MW00416112

Praise for *Skip the Waiting Room*

...king read, *Skip the Waiting Room* offers a visionary look
... is changing the healthcare landscape. The authors
... case for why telemedicine is not just a temporary
...lthcare."

—NATHAN CHAPPELL, AI inventor and
coauthor of *The Generosity Crisis*

...And great need. From an aging
...uggling with substance abuse
...e transformations brought
...think differently to reach
...ilities? How can we do
... those questions and
... The revolution is
...-read this book,

...e *of Values*

...th-
... the
...ually
...ack to

...medicine
...f Medicine

"In just a single decade, fueled by a global pandemic, telemedicine has moved from the fringes to medicine's main stage. Telemedicine is now considered an essential component of health care delivery in almost all practice environments.

The authors, physician entrepreneurs and pioneers in the field, share their own experiences starting and growing a telemedicine practice. Using personal anecdotes and simple vignettes, they illustrate the truly transformative nature of telemedicine.

Despite the many benefits of this powerful new modality of hea[illegible] care delivery for systems and providers, the authors remind us o[illegible] true value of telemedicine—when utilized appropriately, it ac[illegible] helps move the focus of care from institutions and providers b[illegible] the patient, where it belongs."

—**STUART SWADRON,** MD, professor of emergency [illegible] at the Keck School o[illegible]

SKIP THE WAITING ROOM

How Telehealth Will Transform Medicine for Patients and Doctors

CHRIS ROVIN
JARED SHEEHAN
TALIB OMER, MD

with MICHAEL ASHLEY

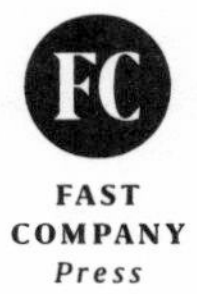

FAST COMPANY *Press*

This book is intended as a reference volume only, not as a medical manual. The information given here is designed to help you make informed decisions about your health. It is not intended as a substitute for any treatment that may have been prescribed by your doctor. If you suspect that you have a medical problem, you should seek competent medical help. You should not begin a new health regimen without first consulting a medical professional.

Fast Company Press
New York, New York
www.fastcompanypress.com

Distributed by Greenleaf Book Group

For ordering information or special discounts for bulk purchases, please contact Greenleaf Book Group at PO Box 91869, Austin, TX 78709, 512.891.6100.

Design and composition by Greenleaf Book Group
Cover design by Greenleaf Book Group
Cover image used under license from ©AdobeStock.com/Digital Bazaar
and ©AdobeStock.com/ST.art

Publisher's Cataloging-in-Publication data is available.

Print ISBN: 978-1-63908-105-9

eBook ISBN: 978-1-63908-106-6

To offset the number of trees consumed in the printing of our books, Greenleaf donates a portion of the proceeds from each printing to the Arbor Day Foundation. Greenleaf Book Group has replaced over 50,000 trees since 2007.

Printed in the United States of America on acid-free paper

24 25 26 27 28 29 30 31 10 9 8 7 6 5 4 3 2 1

First Edition

Contents

Foreword: Bridging the Distance

Telehealth. Telemedicine. What strange words they are! Even to me, a telehealth provider, they conjure up images of *Star Trek*, *The Andromeda Strain*, computers the size of living rooms, robots, and Will Robinson. What, exactly, *is* telehealth, and why should you read about it?

Because, for one, chances are you will be logging in to speak to a telehealth provider sometime in your near future, if you haven't already. Basically, it is the wave of the future of healthcare delivery—well, not just the future but the *present*. And as a likely participant in this form of healthcare, by reading this book, you may gain a better understanding of how it can best serve you.

Unlike any book I've yet encountered about telehealth, it delves into the history of our healthcare model (do not fear, reader; it is a quick and informative rather than tedious journey) and brings us up to speed on how and why we arrived at this landmark in healthcare delivery. It explains not only *what* telehealth is but *why* it is and why it is a good thing for the healthcare consumer. Which is you and me.

As for my take as an emergency physician, I have witnessed rather alarming changes in healthcare delivery happen at an even more alarming rate of speed. What I find a remarkable and unexpected unique quality of telemedicine is its ironic ability to bridge the distance between patient and provider. For too long, the doctor-patient relationship has been skewed to the point where it appears as if the patient works for the doctor, when, of course, the opposite is true. Patients must rearrange their schedules to fit in with those of their doctors instead of the other way around. It is considered normal and acceptable to take a day from work after waiting weeks to months for an appointment, only to be kept for hours in a waiting room. Telemedicine changes this, to the great benefit of patients. Not to mention the benefit for doctors—imagine not being forced to see patients to the point of burnout, to be able to meet both patients' needs *and your own*.

Imagine two people entering a virtual space where they only hear each other's voice, or maybe they see only each other's eyes. No lab coats, no paper robes. Just two people talking about how one can help the other, exchanging information, communicating. Imagine not knowing if the other is rich, poor, well-dressed, liberal, or conservative—just that they're a person, in their office or in their home or on lunchbreak from their job, with their grandchild or new puppy watching closely as you both speak and listen, surprisingly often sharing a laugh or a tear. At the end of it, you, as the doctor, have helped someone. Even if that help is just to assure them that, yes, they do need to go today to the emergency room. And you, as the patient, are now prepared for what to expect when you get there, feeling validation and agency to ask questions and know you deserve thoughtful answers.

Like all good medicine, this book meets the reader where they are and provides a road map to a meaningful conversation between provider and patient. Although much of the book concentrates on patient-centered topics, it also provides valuable insight into the world of healthcare providers. This type of frank, transparent dialog has sadly heretofore been lacking from the industry that has insidiously become our current healthcare model.

So, if you're a doctor who has thought about working in telemedicine, or a patient who thinks telemedicine may be an option for you in the future, this is an excellent primer for what to expect along your travels. Happy reading!

DR. ANNE TINTINALLI,
professor of emergency medicine

PART I

YESTERDAY

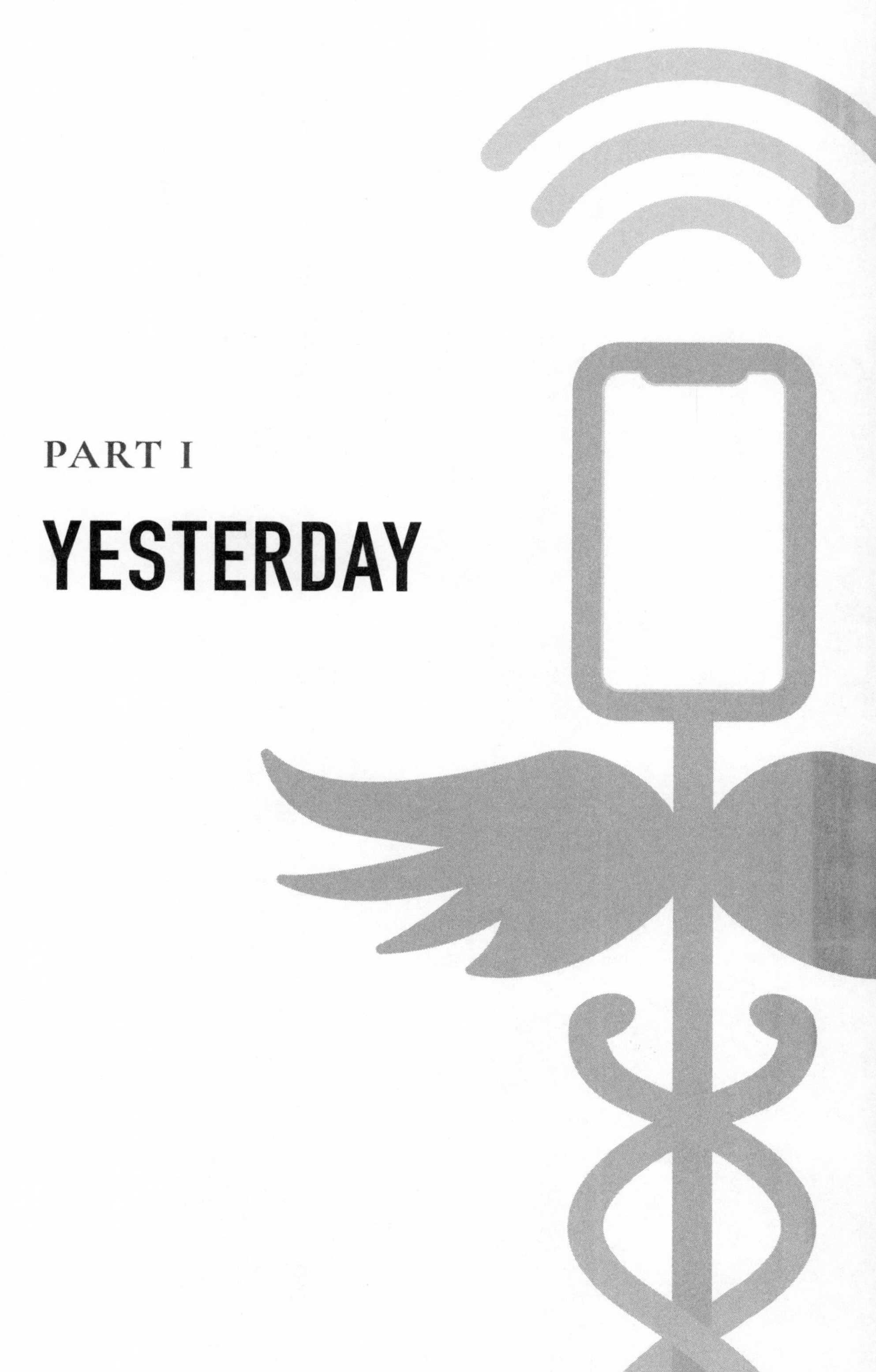

CHAPTER 1

Never Waste a Crisis: The Telehealth Revolution's Time Is Now

March 2020. A man we'll call Simon lives in Orange County, California. He wakes at 2:00 a.m. feeling like a vise is crushing his chest. Weak and lacking energy, he still can't go back to sleep. A nasty cough keeps him up all night.

Early the next morning, he calls his primary care physician, concerned.

"Can you get me in for an appointment?" he asks the dispatcher. "I think I might have COVID."

"I'm sorry. Our office is closed due to shelter-in-place orders."

Fingers to his throbbing temples, Simon groans. "What can I do?"

"You tried the ER?"

Simon pales, his face the image of dread. He pictures a lobby overflowing with dying people, their contorted bodies like something out of a horror flick.

"I—I can't go there."

Things don't improve for Simon that day. Despite taking copious amounts of DayQuil, plus his wife's best efforts to nurse him back to health, his symptoms worsen. Halfway through taking a hot bath the next day, Simon finds he can't breathe. *Don't panic*, he tells himself. *You've got this.*

Only he's not so sure. With his wife, Jane, away with the kids, he's home alone. She won't be back for at least thirty minutes. Grabbing his keys, he stumbles into slippers, heading for his car. His breathing hasn't returned to normal, but it's not as bad. At least he's not gasping for breath as he drives to the ER. Still, he doesn't want to push things by calling Jane.

Exiting his vehicle, Simon stops at the hospital entrance. On the other side of the tinted glass is his nightmare: Sick people. Lots of them. If he doesn't yet have COVID, he definitely will if he enters.

Then something occurs to him.

Years ago, just before their trip to London, Jane saw a doctor online to get medicine for their son. Simon recalls thinking how easy it all was.

He checks his phone. Contact info for the telehealth group is still there. Returning to his car, Simon goes online to book an appointment. To his relief, he gets one immediately with a highly educated physician in Washington state.

"You did the right thing," Dr. Wexler tells him via video chat from Washington as Simon settles back in the car seat. "No need to expose yourself to other at-risk patients."

"Do I have COVID?" Simon cuts to the chase.

"That's impossible for me to tell you without a PCR test. But we can do other things right now. Have you a pulse oximeter?"

"At home."

"Good. As soon as you're back, put it on your finger and read the display. If the number's below 90, that's when you know to return to the ER."

Peering out his windshield, Simon sees a sick man breach the doors, exposing himself to all the other sick people. Simon shudders.

"What should I do in the meantime?"

"Monitor your symptoms. If your body temp goes up or your cough worsens, those are important warning signs."

Simon sighs. "At least there's one good thing. My breath's normal."

Dr. Wexler's easy smile helps relax Simon even more. "That's encouraging. It's gonna be okay. We'll get through this together."

SILVER LINING AMONG DARK CLOUDS

Several years after COVID-19 paralyzed the world, it's easy to forget just how frightened we all were by the novel coronavirus pandemic. Especially back in March 2020 as leaders and medical professionals scrambled to respond. If you take a moment to reflect on how you felt during that time, you might find you shared Simon's deep apprehensions, not only about COVID-19 but about even stepping foot in an ER at the start of the illness hysteria.

There weren't many bright spots in those early pandemic days. The best thing we can say is at least the virus didn't affect our young so severely as many had feared. If it had, the public would have been even more terrified.

The other big impact was widespread adoption of telemedicine, virtual medical consultations over the phone, the internet, or specific collaboration platforms. Prior to COVID-19, this medical approach was not nearly so prevalent in America. We know this personally as the founders of QuickMD, a telehealth platform designed to provide medical services and consultations affordably and digitally. Such service includes virtual visits with healthcare professionals for diagnosis, treatment, and prescriptions. When the COVID-19 pandemic led government regulators to broaden telehealth regulations, QuickMD expanded to become a national provider, catering to patients who previously had limited access to healthcare services.

It's worth briefly describing our background and credentials.

Talib Omer, MD, founded QuickMD in 2019. Driven by entrepreneurial zeal and his experience as an emergency medicine doctor,

Dr. Omer's vision set in motion our company with an emphasis on supporting those who are so often underserved in the market—whether because of financial or geographical constraints. Ever since our inception, Dr. Omer has acted as our captain and organizing force for our ship, steering us ever forward with medical acumen and compassion.

Our chief innovation officer, Jared Sheehan, holds a master of science degree from Johns Hopkins University. Before QuickMD, Jared served as chief executive officer of PwrdBy, a social impact incubator designed to nurture and accelerate innovative nonprofits. As chief operating officer of QuickMD, he spearheaded the TeleMAT (medication-assisted treatment) program, designed to combat the opioid addiction epidemic.

As vice president of operations at QuickMD, Chris Rovin is an expert in transformative healthcare technology. Previously, Chris was foundational in building several other tech companies, including we-search.org and Neeka Health. Beyond managing our staff of healthcare providers at QuickMD, Chris handles processes—everything from marketing to compliance.

Returning to the big picture, COVID-19's effect on telehealth's adoption has been profound, far surpassing initial estimates. According to a study cited in the National Library of Medicine at the National Institutes of Health, the first three months of the pandemic witnessed a staggering 766 percent increase in telemedicine encounters through private insurance claims, with telemedicine's share of all medical interactions soaring from 0.3 percent in the period from March to June 2019 to 23.6 percent for the same months in 2020.[1]

This dramatic shift underscores the rapid pivot toward virtual care as a cornerstone of healthcare delivery. Furthermore, McKinsey and Company's analysis highlights an even more astonishing trend: a whopping 3,800 percent increase in telemedicine utilization when comparing the pre-pandemic period to the post-pandemic reality.[2] These figures not only illustrate the scale of telehealth's integration into the extant healthcare system but also suggest a lasting transformation in how medical care is now accessed and delivered, pointing toward a future where telemedicine plays a more central role in the healthcare ecosystem.

While numerous facilities were closing, an additional invaluable resource was being offered in spring 2020: telemedicine triage. Consider Elmhurst Hospital Center in Queens, New York. "One year ago, the facility was dubbed 'coronavirus ground zero' by one emergency room physician—being the hardest-hit hospital not only in New York City, but in the country," wrote Dr. Alexis E. Carrington for ABC News in a March 2021 piece. "Elmhurst had a patient roster that was over 230% capacity during the last week of February and the first week of March of 2020."[3]

Coauthor Talib Omer, an emergency medicine physician in Los Angeles, had a similar experience. According to him, the early COVID virus was very potent. Patients didn't know if they had the common cold or COVID. The ER was overflowing. Because of this they had to set up tents outside the hospital for triage. Worse, there was so much misinformation that patients didn't know what to believe. In fact, Dr. Omer saw plenty who would have been better off staying home. Likewise, many patients who should have been in the ER thought it would be okay to stay home instead.

Though exact figures have yet to emerge, it's indisputable telemedicine helped contain what could have been a groundswell of even more frightened patients to ERs like his in those perilous early days. Sick with COVID or merely suspecting they were infected, more fearful and uncertain patients would have swamped our already strained healthcare system.

Instead, telemedicine served as a "component of forward triage in a pandemic," according to Vikas Gupta and colleagues: "Based on patient self-reporting, telemedicine potentially prevented face-to-face COVID-related encounters. Patients expressed satisfaction with the virtual process and were less likely to pursue in-person consultation. Leveraging a telehealth strategy for forward triage has the potential to reduce exposures while conserving healthcare resources."[4]

It's been said that pain can be our greatest teacher. A key insight emerged from this devastating public health crisis on that point. Let's explore it.

WHAT WINSTON CHURCHILL CAN TEACH US

With reference to historical tragedies, World War II may stand head and shoulders above the rest. An estimated 70 million people perished in the conflict, mostly civilians. In its aftermath, prescient global leaders sought to not only rebuild countries but to outright prevent the return of another such catastrophe.

Great Britain's prime minister Winston Churchill was one of them. Reeling from the carnage, he helped form the United Nations to this end and is famously credited with saying, "Never let a good crisis go to waste."[5] Though the COVID-19 pandemic did not kill nearly as many as World War II, it undeniably produced tremendous human misery and anguish on every continent save Antarctica. Thus, it's an outsized tragedy with undeniable comparisons.

For our purposes, the key lesson is to seize this moment to not only rebuild healthcare but outright prevent further suffering and needless deaths in a public health crisis. As mentioned, before COVID-19, telemedicine was not widely used in the United States. But now that so many of us have reached out for it like a life preserver to a drowning swimmer, we appreciate its utility. Emerging from our crisis, let's use it to offer better healthcare to far more people.

This is the promise of our book.

A famous saying goes, "Luck occurs when preparation meets inspiration." Whether you believe in such an idea, the scourge of COVID undeniably offers us a chance to do better—to get "lucky." It also allows us to finally address systemic medical problems that might have simply continued if not for such a terrible catalyst. Put another way, the pages to come serve as a primer for those wishing to make refreshing lemonade from so many bitter lemons.

More on those lemons in a moment. For now, it's worth stating who this book is for. Though we all should care about health as mortal creatures with physical bodies, this content is especially geared to these groups:

- Medical entrepreneurs
- Health leaders
- Business investors
- Patients
- Doctors

Later in the chapter, we explain why all these stakeholders should care about this content. For now, let's take a brief trip down memory lane. Specifically, let's ask the following question: Long before anyone encountered COVID, what was healthcare like? (Spoiler alert: not good.)

A BRIEF HISTORY OF MEDICINE

Though official records don't exist for prehistoric times, we have some idea of what medicine was like for our prehistoric ancestors. *Medical News Today* suggests our forebears believed in both natural and supernatural treatments and causes.

> Nobody knows precisely what prehistoric peoples knew about how the human body works, but we can base some guesses on limited evidence that anthropologists have found.
>
> Prehistoric burial practices, for example, suggest that people knew something about bone structure. Scientists have found bones that were stripped of the flesh, bleached, and piled together, according to what part of the body they came from.
>
> There is also archeological evidence that some prehistoric communities practiced cannibalism. These people must have known about the inner organs and where there is most lean tissue or fat in the human body.[6]

Taking a leap from such grisly anthropophagy, our journey through the medical ages swiftly advances to the 400s BC, marking the era of Hippocrates in ancient Greece. Renowned as the father of modern medicine, Hippocrates was instrumental in shaping our contemporary understanding of health. He asserted that diseases stem from natural causes and, accordingly, can be treated via natural means, famously stating, "Natural forces within us are the true healers of disease."[7] His contributions weren't limited to his well-known oath, either; rather, they laid the foundational principles for medical ethics and practice. However, during his time, the concept of professional accreditation was nonexistent, allowing anyone to proclaim themselves as a doctor. According to *World History Encyclopedia*, doctors in the ancient world relied heavily on astrology, divination, and omens.[8]

This meant all kinds of nasty procedures could be applied in the service of health by (often unwitting) healers. Here's a fun one: trepanation. According to *History*, "Humanity's oldest form of surgery is also one of its most gruesome. As far back as 7,000 years ago, civilizations around the world engaged in trepanation—the practice of boring holes in the skull as a means of curing illnesses. Researchers can only speculate on how or why this form of brain surgery first developed."[9] Side note: The late neuroscientist Charles Gross reported that this practice continued as late as the 1800s in Central America, where "the survival rate from trephining (and many other operations) rarely reached 10 percent."[10]

Our narrative progresses from there to a significant milestone in the evolution of healthcare with the establishment of the first documented general hospital in the early ninth century around 805 AD, in Baghdad. This development signified a pivotal shift from the earlier, simpler facilities catering to the ill with minimal organization and rudimentary care. These institutions, while existing in various forms since antiquity, were fundamentally transformed in Baghdad, leading to the complex and structured hospital systems we recognize today. This reality reflects the sophisticated approach to healthcare and medical ethics that emerged from the Islamic world, underscoring diverse contributions to the medical field across cultures and epochs.

So were the Middle Ages better medically? You probably know the answer. No. Few doctors existed in western Europe between 500 AD and 1500 AD. That's largely because training could take years. There weren't many universities to convey such knowledge. Plus, you had to be able to read, write, and decipher Latin—a nonstarter for much of the population struggling to survive.

Perhaps the biggest problem in medieval Europe was that medical authorities lacked an understanding of germs, antiseptics, and anesthetics. Instead, many subscribed to Hippocrates's erroneous views on the four humors as the central cause for health problems. Galen, a second-century Roman doctor to various emperors, later expanded on the four humors, leading it to become a widespread theory.

Say what you will about the humors—and we will momentarily—Galen's findings on them were at least *backed by what we now know as the scientific method* (although this term had yet to be coined). That's because Galen gleaned his insights from dissecting animals to better know how to treat humans. Unfortunately, Galen also believed in the mistaken notion that four humors—or liquids (phlegm, blood, yellow bile, black bile)—were responsible for determining one's health or the lack thereof.

According to an article published by the BBC:

> If the humours stayed in balance then a person remained healthy, but if there was too much of one humour then illness occurred.
>
> - If a patient had a runny nose, it was because of an excess of phlegm in the body.
> - If a patient had nose bleeds, it was because of an excess of blood.[11]

It was important to keep the patient's body in balance. This was done by removing excess fluid. The most common method used by doctors in the Middle Ages was bloodletting.

Unfamiliar with bloodletting? Here's *Healthline*'s description of the once popular medical practice:

> Bloodletting was the name given to the removal of blood for medical treatment. It was believed to rid the body of impure fluids to cure a host of conditions. Originally, bloodletting involved cutting a vein or artery—typically at the elbow or knee—to remove the affected blood. Over time, specialized instruments and techniques—including the use of leeches—were developed to make more precise cuts and improve control over how much blood was removed. Blood was typically drained until you passed out, which for most people amounted to about 20 ounces of blood.[12]

Bloodletting was done in many cultures, not just in western Europe, through the Middle Ages up through the early modern period.

But as morbid as these treatments were, and flawed as our medical understandings were back then, the early modern era (roughly 1500–1800) wasn't much better, healthwise. In fact, as late as the mid- to late 1800s (post–Industrial Revolution), European and American hospitals were cesspools of disease and death. Hold this picture in your mind: filthy nineteenth-century hospitals. Now recall that a crisis would one day emerge that would confer an opportunity for positive medical change (to paraphrase Churchill a century later). That crisis/opportunity for nineteenth-century America was the Civil War (1861–1865). "The Civil War proved to be a catalyst in advancing 19th century medicine," according to Battlefields.org. Here's how:

> Lacking sufficient supplies and knowledge, both armies struggled to control the emergence of various diseases such as measles, smallpox, and typhoid. At the beginning of the war, germ theory, antiseptic practices (sterilizing instruments and wearing gloves), and effective hospital systems were virtually nonexistent. As a result of poor sanitation, diet, ventilation, and bad hygiene, disease and infection spread rampant, making disease more deadly than the battle wounds experienced on the field.[13]

Fortunately, all those filthy hospitals riddled with screaming amputees and overrun with staph infections gave way to the modern, sanitary medical conditions we expect in today's facilities. At least in the United States. With such tremendous—*and desperately needed*—healthcare advances came reduced mortality rates, especially among children, infants and new mothers, leading to longer lives and better health outcomes.

ONE LAST STOP

We now conclude our historical tour with one more crucial antecedent that has special bearing on the present. Decades after hospitals adopted contemporary hygienic medical care practices (such as washing hands between patients, using disinfectants, and other advances that included antibiotics)—yet still before today's era—doctors made house calls.

The house call—physicians visiting patients in their homes—was a mid-century standard. According to *U.S. News and World Report*, "In 1930, about 40 percent of doctor-patient interactions were through house calls." This same article elaborates on the benefits of this personalized arrangement. "From a patient's perspective, summoning a doctor to your house has plenty of appeal: No waiting rooms, traffic or skipped work. No dragging a sick and tired body out of bed to see a doctor whose prescription is to go back to bed. No feeling like a number."[14]

Also, because a major focus of our book concerns not just fixing how we deliver care, but also how we improve conditions for providers, it's worth mentioning how this previous model helped the latter. Again, we turn to the same article, "For doctors, aspects of the practice are attractive too: more satisfying patient interaction and the ability to see how patients live."[15]

WHY SHOULD YOU CARE?

Beyond the fact that you (presumably) have a body and are subject to the same diseases, ailments, accidents, and the like that have afflicted humanity for millennia, there are other, more tangible reasons to read on. Following are the main reasons why this issue especially matters to the healthcare marketplace.

Reason 1: Like It or Not, the Telehealth Revolution Is Happening

Did you know hospitals are closing in record numbers? In 2021, Sidecar Health reported the following: "Since 2005, 181 rural hospitals have shut their doors. The causes are many: an older, poorer population; advances in outpatient medical procedures; and more recently, a decision among many Southern states against expanding Medicaid under the Patient Protection and Affordable Care Act, aka ACA."[16]

This problem isn't limited to isolated communities. As NPR reported in September 2020, "While rural hospitals have been closing at a quickening pace over the past two decades, a number of inner-city hospitals now face a similar fate. And experts fear that the economic damage inflicted by the COVID-19 pandemic on safety net hospitals and the ailing finances of the cities and states that subsidize them are helping push some urban hospitals over the edge."[17]

This bad news couldn't come at a worse time. As the *Hill* reported one year before the pandemic, in 2019, "The average American is getting older as baby boomers hit retirement age and natural births decrease, according to new data from the U.S. Census Bureau."[18] So many closures restricting medical access will especially hit seniors hard, the demographic likeliest to require care. Telehealth, on the other hand, holds the promise to course-correct our ever-dwindling numbers of facilities and physician shortages, major problems affecting an increasingly aging population. Telehealth is no silver bullet. But it does provide significant benefits that have already been accepted—and embraced—by millions in the last few years.

Reason 2: This Is a Big Opportunity for All of Us

Reflecting on Simon's narrative, it's easy to empathize with his predicament. Many of us have encountered the frustration of being unable to access timely medical care, whether for ourselves or for our loved ones, and understand the distress it can cause. This situation is further exacerbated by the escalating crisis of prolonged wait times for outpatient appointments, increasingly acknowledged as a significant public health concern.

Recent reports, such as one by Connecticut Public Radio, indicate that the average wait time to see a new physician has reached 26 days, with even longer delays in certain specialties.[19] For instance, securing an OB-GYN appointment can now take as long as 31.4 days, a 19 percent increase since 2017, as detailed by *STAT*.[20] Wait times have also significantly increased across dermatology, cardiology, and orthopedic surgery specialties, highlighting the critical need to address this bottleneck in healthcare delivery.

In this context, telehealth emerges as a significant improvement, promising to transform our challenged healthcare system. By harnessing technology, telehealth is poised to drastically reduce these wait times, providing patients with quicker access to care that's both compassionate and dignified. This represents an essential opportunity for all of us to leverage the advantages of telehealth, not merely as a matter of convenience but as an imperative step forward in achieving better health outcomes for all.

In a related point, as Craig Guillot, writing for *HealthTech*, explains, "The pandemic has highlighted existing racial, economic, and geographic disparities that can hinder access to medical treatment, according to the *American Journal of Managed Care*. A rapid shift to telehealth could improve access for marginalized groups faced with the double challenge of limited resources and poor connectivity."[21]

Even better, telehealth promises to positively change how we deliver care. In short, we stand to become a much healthier society in several important ways. Following are a few:

- Greater access to (nonlocal) physicians, including specialists and subspecialists
- More flexibility with scheduling virtual visits
- Reduced need to commute to appointments
- Ability to monitor health better remotely and in real time
- Prevention of exposure to infectious diseases
- Lower costs due to reduced overhead for practices
- Shorter wait times for appointments, streamlining the process and improving patient satisfaction

Reason 3: This Is a Big Opportunity for You

Remember Blockbuster? How about Kodak? Both of these once successful companies failed to see life's one inescapable truth: the only constant is change. What works today is not guaranteed tomorrow. Returning to reason 1, the telehealth train has left the station. The genie is out of the bottle.

The American public has now had three years to get used to this medical delivery model. Most patients utilizing telemedicine services report being satisfied, according to the *International Journal of Environmental Research and Public Health*.[22] It's hard for them to imagine going back. At least this is the prognosis of a December 2020 *Harvard Business Review* article by Jessica Dudley and Iyue Sung. They write that their survey patients were just as likely—or even slightly *more* likely—to rate their care providers highly after telemedicine visits than after visits they had to make in person. This held true across medical specialties.[23]

Now back to Blockbuster and Kodak. These companies once thrived as giants on the business stage. Their very names were synonymous with success. These days? Their failures are cautionary tales, offering warnings to other companies—and industries—reluctant to shift with the times. They show us the truth behind innovation and capitalism. There will be winners and losers in the coming years.

Who are most poised to benefit from this medical care disruption?

- Those who comply with (changing) laws
- Those who rapidly adapt to dynamic conditions
- Those who identify health areas most likely to benefit from telemedicine

This final consideration takes us to our next topic.

AREAS TO WATCH

It would be foolish to think the telemedicine health model will fully replace current healthcare delivery. It's not feasible—or advisable—to recommend the distanced option to a woman in labor. Or to her husband suffering a heart attack.

Telehealth has its limitations. To bring it back to Simon, our stand-in for so many patients exploring this care model, should he have had a knife wound or a gunshot wound, it would be absurd to imagine him booking an online appointment to handle his emergency.

This leads us to an important question: Which medical specialties are best suited for telehealth? In our assessment, those specialties lending themselves most naturally to telemedicine are those that do not rely heavily on procedures, intensive monitoring, frequent laboratory testing, extensive physical exams, or comprehensive multispecialty care. However, most specialties can reap the benefits of telehealth, albeit with a few exceptions. These are the areas we believe are suited for telehealth, along with some specific use examples for each:

Behavioral Health

- Addiction
- Depression/anxiety
- Family and marriage counseling
- Adolescent challenges
- Obsessive-compulsive disorders/attention-deficit/hyperactivity disorder
- Conduct disorder
- Sexual compulsion
- Codependency

Acute or Urgent Care

- Common colds
- Respiratory issues like colds, the flu, and COVID-19
- Constipation
- Nausea/diarrhea
- Prescription medication fill and refill
- Bronchitis or cough
- Rashes or skin problems/minor allergies
- Urinary tract or bladder infection
- Headaches, back or muscle pain
- Pink eye

Sexual Health

- Sexually transmitted diseases
- Reproductive and fertility concerns

- Prenatal and postpartum concerns
- Erectile dysfunctionality
- Menopause/women's health

Proactive Health and Wellness

- Ongoing prevention and optimization
- Wearables for real-time tracking/testing/monitoring
- Optimizing nutrition
- Diet and weight loss

Specialist Care

- Severe allergies
- Gerontology
- Gastroenterology
- Aspects of ear, nose, throat (ENT) treatment
- Aspects of oncology
- Surgery follow-ups
- Second opinion (multiple specialties)
- End-of-life care

Conversely, there are medical specialties completely inappropriate for telemedicine. An exhaustive list is impossible; let's cover some major areas.

While telemedicine offers extensive benefits across various medical specialties, there are certain areas where its applicability is more limited or nuanced. It's important to recognize that while telemedicine cannot replace in-person care in some scenarios, it can still play a supportive role. The following list outlines major areas where telemedicine is not the primary mode of care, highlighting how it can nonetheless complement traditional medical practices. This is not an exhaustive list, but it provides perspective on the balanced role of telehealth in the broader healthcare landscape.

- *Emergency room care*. An example is immediate care for accidents or critical illnesses (e.g., car accidents). However, follow-up consultations or post-emergency care can be managed through telehealth.
- *Surgery*. For example, performing surgeries like Lasik remotely is not feasible. However, telemedicine can be valuable for presurgical consultations and post-operative follow-ups.
- *Giving birth*. For example, direct assistance during childbirth, such as a doula's physical support, cannot be replaced by telehealth. However, pre-labor consultations and postpartum care can be effectively conducted via telehealth.
- *High-acuity cases*. Examples are conditions requiring constant intensive care, such as life-threatening illnesses. However, telehealth can be used for remote monitoring and consultations related to these conditions.
- *Hospice care*. An example is direct end-of-life care, which often requires a physical presence. However, telehealth can facilitate consultations with family members and provide psychological support.
- *Rare diseases*. Examples include complex cases such as acquired aplastic anemia, requiring specialized in-person care.

However, initial consultations and follow-up care can benefit from telemedicine, especially in reaching specialists.

- *Chemotherapy*. Intravenous chemotherapy is administered in-person. However, remote telehealth can support pre- and post-treatment consultations, including oral chemotherapy management.
- *Most controlled substance prescriptions*. An example is prescribing powerful drugs that have a high risk of misuse. However, telemedicine can be used for initial assessments, follow-ups, and monitoring. Still, actual prescriptions might require in-person visits.

Table 1 offers a good starting point for differentiation. On the left are procedures requiring the physical presence of a caregiver and patient. On the right, we list ways in which telehealth could nonetheless provide significant medical value.

Table 1. Telemedicine and in-person cases

Requires in-person visit	Can use telehealth
Surgery	Before-and-after consults
Emergency situation (e.g., gunshot wound)	Before-and-after consults
Labor and delivery/childbirth	Before-and-after consults
High acuity (example: dialysis)	Related consults
Hospice	Consults with family
Rare diseases	Before-and-after consults
Chemotherapy	Before-and-after consults
Specific controlled substance prescriptions	Before-and-after consults

SIX PILLARS FOR TRANSFORMATIVE CARE

Rounding out our discussion, telehealth offers the best option for medical care if at least one or more of the following conditions are present.

1. *Enables greater access:* The increased pool of providers offers more availability to care for the patient. For example, instead of waiting three months to book an allergy specialist, a mother can lock in an appointment online in minutes.
2. *Promotes better patient compliance and follow-up:* The telehealth delivery model can result in higher patient adherence rates. For example, a construction worker with a busy schedule can better follow through with his caregiver's treatment plan as it fits his unique schedule.
3. *Desired care exceeds need:* It is just as possible to provide a better health outcome in a remote setting. Example: a pediatric patient with irritable bowel syndrome (IBS) who spends five hours in an emergency room surrounded by sick people only to receive simple pediatric gas relief medication.
4. *Removes barriers:* It eliminates needless obstacles to being seen by a caregiver. Example: A patient who lives in rural Montana and must drive an hour to see her therapist.
5. *Expedites care:* It speeds up medical treatment without incurring negative effects. Example: A woman with a splitting migraine needn't spend her Saturday night in an urgent care center just to get her migraine prescription filled.
6. *Enables wellness:* It empowers patients to optimize their health without negative consequences. Example: The overweight person who creates a unique diet with his doctor, leading to healthy weight loss.

All six of these pillars show how telemedicine can improve health outcomes for patients. Even better, this model provides benefits to caregivers. Let's now explore how it can help both parties in greater detail.

Pillar 1: Increased Pool of Potential Providers

The best result of our legacy healthcare system is one in which we can find a good doctor in our local area. But this approach is limited by geography. What if you don't live close to any good providers? Telemedicine can reduce this inequity. Removing location constraints, telemedicine makes it easier for a patient to be connected to the correct specialist.

Example patient benefit: A mom in rural Iowa can access an accomplished applied behavior analysis (ABA) specialist in metropolitan Chicago to assess whether her toddler has autism.

Example doctor benefit: A family physician with limited prospects in her remote hometown is freed from applying for positions in her local area. Instead, she can pursue exciting opportunities in diverse regions.

Pillar 2: Higher Patient Compliance and Follow-Up Rates

Too often, medical treatments fail because patients don't follow through on their doctor's plan. Whether it involves taking antibiotics for the right number of days or making a diet change, sometimes patients don't see things through to the end. One reason why? Follow-up appointments are easy to miss. Patients who are feeling better may even cancel them, especially because of their busy lives, inclement weather, or traffic.

Example patient benefit: When a follow-up occurs at home, the patient is more likely to make their appointments and stay on track with treatment(s).

Example doctor benefit: This gives the doctor more assurance that his patients will receive the follow-up needed after they are sent home.

Pillar 3: Desired Care Exceeds the Need

Many families have been there. A child is sick and crying, so the parents take their child to the ER for a minor malady. This is often to secure treatment and relief before the pediatrician's office opens or the next appointment is available (sometimes weeks in the future). Though a common situation, it reveals an inefficiency of our legacy healthcare system. Sometimes we desire a level (or speed) of care that brick-and-mortar doctor's offices can't provide, so we seek alternatives like the ER. This problem compounds in healthcare deserts (areas where facilities are lacking). Telemedicine can eliminate such inefficiencies by providing (close to) immediate appointments with providers around the clock.

Example patient benefit: No need to take off work for a quick five-minute post-op surgery consultation. Instead, a patient can hop on a teleconference with her caregiver to ensure everything is healing properly.

Example doctor benefit: Doctors can stack their appointments, better managing their work-life balance, which may reduce burnout.

Pillar 4: Removing Needless Barriers

Technology is at its best when it removes needless hindrances and makes positive connections. In the future, telemedicine patients can learn more about potential doctors before ever meeting them. Sometimes, understanding who a caregiver is and where they come from makes all the difference for a patient hesitant to seek treatment.

Example patient benefit: Forget about having to see the only marriage therapist in town—because they are the only marriage therapist in town. Instead, a patient can widen their search across the United States.

Example doctor benefit: A doctor wants to treat opioid addiction but worries he can't because it would mean taking a financial gamble on opening a clinic. Instead, he can gain the necessary licensing to provide addiction treatment by partnering with a telehealth provider.

Pillar 5: Expediting Care without Negative Effects

We're a society used to same-day delivery and instant access. That expectation makes it more jarring when we call our doctor's office only to learn there are no appointments available. For weeks. Or months. Just as telemedicine breaks down barriers, increasing the pool of available physicians, it also expedites care. Even so, quicker care is only a positive if it adheres to the highest standards of professionalism.

Example patient benefit: Many telehealth services operate twenty-four hours a day. "Sick call" hours are 24/7. That means a patient can receive expedited care and feel better faster most any time of day.

Example doctor benefit: Flexible schedules and the ability to cover odd hours or overnight shifts especially help doctors with young families.

Pillar 6: Enabling Health Optimization without Harmful Impact

Telemedicine's future is in enabling health optimization. Much like the recent trend in concierge medicine (membership-based healthcare), remotely delivered care enables us to become—and stay—healthier. How? Through an ongoing relationship with a doctor emphasizing *wellness*, not just treating a particular issue. Health optimization is a realistic option for even *more* people when it includes the cost effectiveness and efficiency of telemedicine baked into it.

Example patient benefit: A corporate executive wants to be healthier, but she works long hours, and she recently had a baby. She needn't sacrifice wellness on the altar of work or family. Instead, she gets to schedule wellness appointments.

Example doctor benefit: Telemedicine can improve health outcomes by changing the role of doctors from caregivers to care enablers, helping them achieve their professional purpose.

If all this sounds too good to be true, that's probably because the inertia of our legacy model has conditioned both patients and caregivers to believe what we've got is the best we can do. It's not. Not by a long shot, as this chapter demonstrates. But before we delve further into how telehealth will vastly improve how doctors deliver care, we must air some pent-up grievances. It's time to learn why the waiting room experience hasn't been working for anyone.

Not even doctors.

CHAPTER 2

Waiting Rooms Haven't Been Working—for Anyone

There's a telling cold open from the hit series *Seinfeld* in which comedian Jerry Seinfeld riffs on an all-too-common phenomenon. "Waiting room. I hate when they make you wait in the room. 'Cause it says: *waiting room*. There's no chance of *not* waiting. 'Cause they call it . . . 'the waiting room.' They're gonna use it. They got it. It's all set up for you to wait."[1]

Seinfeld goes on to describe the frustrating process you know well if you've visited a doctor anytime in the last 40 years. Sound familiar? Upon signing in with reception, you must sit there with a magazine or book (nowadays you can at least go on your phone) and wait. *Interminably*. Or at least until someone finally pops in with a chart and calls your name.

"You kinda look around at the other people in the room," says Seinfeld, describing this moment. "Well, I guess I've been chosen. I'll see you all later."

Then you scamper off with the nurse. But your wait isn't over. Instead, you're only taken to the *next* waiting room. This one's smaller. And usually less stocked with old *Highlights* and *People* issues. It comes equipped with tongue depressors and other medical accoutrements. Here you shall wait some more. And why not? After all, that's the name of this place.

POSTMORTEM

What a hassle. Think about all that time wasted for you, the patient. You spend time researching the doctor you're there to see. You spend time on the phone or online scheduling the day's visit. Then you spend the time required to request an hour or two off work for your appointment. Plus, you spend time arranging your schedule to take that time off.

When the big day arrives, you then spend the time needed to commute to the brick-and-mortar building. This could require several hours, especially if you live in a rural area or a large city like Chicago or Los Angeles. Also, if you do have kids, coordinating schedules with your spouse, partner, or babysitter adds to the overall time commitment. Then you spend time parking. Upon arriving at your appointment, whether for primary care or a specialist visit, waiting is often an inevitable part of the experience.

The duration of this wait can vary significantly. For instance, primary care appointments might have shorter wait times, but specialty consultations, urgent care visits, and emergency department trips can involve much longer waits. It's important to recognize that these wait times can be quite variable and context dependent. And again, they are just *one* aspect of the overall time investment required for in-person medical visits.

By contrast, the average time a customer waits to receive fast food is five minutes. An upscale restaurant will typically serve you in 10 to 15 minutes.

To make matters worse, wait times have *increased* over the years. In

2016, CNBC referenced a new survey recording "that the vast majority of patients—85 percent—say they have to wait anywhere from 10 minutes to 30 minutes past their scheduled appointment time to actually see their doctor."[2] Note: This doesn't count the time for scheduling and coordinating one's appointment.

But that's not all. "New research published in the *American Journal of Managed Care* estimates that, on average, it takes 121 minutes each time a person seeks medical care. The total includes 37 minutes of travel time, as well as 87 minutes at the doctor's office or clinic," according to *Money*. Unfortunately, you as the patient can only expect to be seen for about 20 minutes. "The other hour or so tends to be spent doing paperwork, communicating with non-medical office staff, and just plain sitting around waiting."[3] More on this in a moment.

For now, as the saying goes, time is money. And there are real costs for patients who must wait around to see their caregiver. In a report by NBC News referencing a previous study, researchers estimated that the average American incurs a loss of nearly $50 per doctor's visit in terms of opportunity costs, not including the fee for services. The article highlights that people "spent more than two hours on the average doctor's visit," losing that work time at an average $43 in lost productivity. This was more than the average out-of-pocket cost of $32.[4] Note that because these figures are from 2015, given the rate of inflation and changes in the healthcare landscape since then, the actual costs today are likely to be significantly higher.

But that's not all the deleterious consequences. The waiting room experience especially harms one specific American demographic. According to NBC News, minorities wait for care longer than other populations. Citing a letter published by researchers in *JAMA Internal Medicine*, NBC News reports that "Black, Hispanic, and unemployed people spent 25 percent to 28 percent longer on medical visits."[5]

These statistics are bad enough. But let's not forget all the self-employed people in this nation. Unlike many of their W2 counterparts, they cannot request paid leave from their employer to visit a doctor. Instead, and especially if they own and operate a small business requiring their presence, any time lost can be a stiff financial hardship.

Imagine you own a solo food truck operation in Austin, Texas. If you don't come in to work that day to prepare food for your customers, no employer or fellow employee will be there to pick up the slack for you. No one will cover your shift. You will simply be out the money you didn't earn that day because you had to take yourself or your sick child to urgent care.

Now, let's take this scenario a bit further. Returning to our Austin-based food truck vendor, what if instead of having a sick child who needs to see a doctor just one time for a cold, let's imagine this child required *multiple* doctor visits. Consider what would happen if this child had a chronic condition like multiple sclerosis, diabetes, or cancer, requiring extensive treatment. Each time our food truck entrepreneur had to take their sick child to the doctor, it would cost them dearly.

Here are but a few of the ways:

- Fuel costs
- Lost revenue for lost work hours
- Insurance premiums
- Out-of-pocket expenses
- Parking charges

To add insult to injury, it's not uncommon for overworked doctors and their equally stressed staff to cancel appointments at the last minute or to make patients wait way past the typical expected length.

Especially if they are overbooked and/or short-staffed. Some frustrated self-employed people have even gone so far as to charge their doctors for wasting their time.

That's precisely what writer Susan Perry explains in an opinion piece for *MinnPost*. She begins by describing waiting in an ophthalmologist's office once for more than 90 minutes. What especially annoyed her was the unspoken assumption that the doctor's time was more valuable than her own. "I never thought to send the doctor a bill for the wages I lost during that wasted hour in her waiting room. I didn't know I could." She didn't take matters into her own hands that day, but she understands patients who do, including one owner of a California public relations firm, who "told *MedPage Today* reporter Kristina Flore that she billed her ophthalmologist . . . for making her wait 45 minutes past her appointment time."[6]

If waiting to see clinic doctors is a hassle, ER wait times are worse. Using data extracted between January 2020 and March 2021, Becker's compiled average emergency room wait times. North Dakota represents the lowest end at 104 minutes. Meanwhile, Maryland residents, on the far extreme of the spectrum, can expect to wait 228 minutes.[7] To understand why these waits are so lengthy, we turn to Hippo Reads for a breakdown.

> Waits and delays are common in ERs across the United States, and, according to the CDC, they're increasing. Hospitals with sufficient funding have responded by adding more beds and hiring more staff—yet the problem persists. To a certain extent, the problem's persistence makes sense. ER visits aren't scheduled and are unpredictable. Patients with and without insurance rely on the emergency department as a source of primary care, so they are often overcrowded. In this system, perhaps waits, delays, and cancellations are inevitable.[8]

Anyone who has spent time in an ER knows exactly what this is like. It feels as if these statistics *understate* the issue. Coauthor Michael Ashley can recall spending more than three hours at an emergency room in Mission Viejo, California, waiting to see a doctor for his sick infant one weekend when all the urgent care facilities were closed. And the county hospital's emergency department of coauthor Dr. Omer routinely has 15- to 20-hour wait times—on some days even up to 30 hours.

On a national level, the situation in emergency rooms has become increasingly challenging. In 2019, KFF reported a notable trend in California: a growing number of emergency room patients are opting to leave crowded hospitals before ever being seen by a healthcare provider.

> About 352,000 California ER visits in 2017 ended when patients left after seeing a doctor but before their medical care was complete. That's up by 57%, or 128,000 incidents, from 2012, according to data from the Office of Statewide Health Planning and Development. Another 322,000 would-be patients left the emergency room without seeing a doctor, up from 315,000 such episodes in 2012.[9]

Now consider the Loftons. In 2021, the family waited in a Memphis, Tennessee, hospital for *50 hours* for treatment. (An older Lofton came to the Methodist South Hospital in Whitehaven complaining of a serious infection in her legs. Since she couldn't be seen by any urgent care facilities in the area, her family was forced to wait with her in shifts for the more than two days she spent there.) Egregious as this example might seem on its face, even this lengthy wait time is sadly not such an anomaly for Shelby County, Tennessee, where it occurred.

Covering this story for WREG, Shay Arthur reports, "Shelby

County's Health Department Director is saying she too has received reports of long ER wait times." The report states that the time frames range from 36 to as high as 60 hours, according to Dr. Michelle Taylor, director of the Shelby County Health Department, at a task force briefing.[10]

Also, just to show this problem is prevalent in all of North America, in 2023, an 86-year-old woman died in an emergency room near Quebec City in Canada after a seven-hour wait. As CTV News Montreal reports, Gilberte Gosselin entered the Hôtel-Dieu hospital in Lévis for a hip fracture. After undergoing hospital tests, she was first told she required surgery. Instead, her condition worsened to the point even this would not be enough to stabilize her condition.

She was then supposed to be transferred to another room for end-of-life care. "Instead, Gosselin stayed in the hallway of the emergency room, where she died Thursday morning. Her family says she spent 48 hours in the emergency department without food or water."[11]

Sadly, Gosselin's tale is no outlier.

More patients than you might think have died waiting to be seen in the emergency room. In early 2020, Tashonna Ward, a 25-year-old Wisconsin woman, passed away from an enlarged heart after a prolonged ER wait. According to CBS News, Tashonna Ward lost consciousness after waiting several hours with her sister in Froedtert Hospital after a preliminary chest X-ray and no admittance. Ward could not be revived by paramedics after her sister attempted to drive her, still unconscious, to another facility.[12]

Research also sheds light on the critical impact of wait times in emergency rooms on patient mortality. A striking finding from UPI indicates that as wait times increase, so does the risk of death. "When the wait times rose to between six and eight hours, the death rate was 8% higher than expected, while waiting eight to 12 hours the death rate was 10% higher than expected, compared with patients who were moved along within six hours. That meant an additional person died for every 82 patients delayed for six to eight hours."[13] This statistic underscores the vital importance of reducing wait times in emergency settings to improve patient outcomes.

While death is the most extreme outcome from care delays, many more patients experience poor medical outcomes because of overworked staff. This presents another challenge: poor medical outcomes due to strained caregivers who cannot possibly meet patient demand.

MORE NEGATIVES

Setting aside the issue of overcrowded ER facilities, it's tempting to think that even when you finally arrive at your doctor's office, after all the time coordinating your appointment, taking time off work, getting a babysitter for the kids, navigating through traffic, sourcing a parking spot, then waiting in the big waiting room, then a smaller waiting room, and finally—*finally*—seeing your doctor, you'll receive great care.

You would be wrong.

Christine Sinsky and colleagues conducted a study of 57 family medical physicians to discern how much of their doctor's time went to interacting with them. The research team observed caregivers for 430 hours, assessing how much of their time was spent on four activities:

1. Direct clinical face-to-face time
2. Chart review, ordering of tests, documentation in the electronic health record (EHR), and desk work
3. Administrative tasks
4. Self-reported after-hours work

Here's what they found:

> During the office day, physicians spent 27.0% of their total time on direct clinical face time with patients and 49.2% of their time on EHR and desk work. While in the examination room with patients, physicians spent 52.9% of the time on direct clinical face time and 37.0% on EHR and desk work. The 21 physicians who completed after-hours diaries reported 1 to 2 hours of after-hours work each night, devoted mostly to EHR tasks.[14]

What jumps out at us from reading this study is how limited visits are with providers. After all that waiting to be seen, the average doctor spends only about 27 percent of their time with a patient. Is it believable this abridged sliver will suffice to successfully diagnose and treat someone? Beyond the sheer amount of time wasted in this subpar process, there are other undesirable aspects of the waiting room we have come to know. And loathe.

Here's our top-10 list:

Top 10 Things Patients Resent about the Waiting Room Experience

1. Many waiting rooms send the same offensive message to patients: your time is not important. Or at least not as important as your doctor's.
2. Many are cheerless places with terrible Muzak, dispiriting generic art prints, outdated magazines, and TVs set to one (very loud) channel.
3. Even after you arrive, you can't just see your doctor. Instead, you're told to fill out more paperwork (beyond what you may have completed before arrival).

4. There is a significant chance of contracting an infectious disease from being stuck in a room with ill people for an extended period.
5. There's little to no privacy. Expect to be seen by a slew of other patients and their friends/families who may know you outside of this experience.
6. If you complain about the long wait or other inconvenient aspects of your visit, you can expect little to change. If anything, the staff might opt to move another (less vocal) patient to the head of the line.
7. Often if you need to cancel your appointment at the last minute, even because you're sick and you don't want to infect anyone, you can still expect to be charged for the visit.
8. Unless you brought a book or your phone, there's little else to do while you wait and suffer.
9. The uncertainty and lack of communication about wait times can be distressing, with the anticipation sometimes being worse than knowing the actual duration of the wait.
10. Even after you've been seen by your doctor, the work is not over. Now you must take your prescription to a pharmacy, where you can expect to wait some more or, in numerous cases, the pharmacy refuses to fill it or insurance denies the prescription.

Now that we have analyzed the challenges facing the waiting room from the patient's perspective, it's important to approach the issue from a broader viewpoint within the healthcare system. Medical care involves a complex network of contributors including, but not limited to, patients, doctors, nursing staff, nursing assistants, respiratory therapists, payers, and other healthcare professionals. With this diverse array of stakeholders, a question arises: Is the waiting room functioning effectively for *all* parties involved, particularly healthcare providers? To explore this, let's consider a day in the life of our coauthor, offering insights into the experience from the provider's perspective.

DR. TALIB OMER'S STORY

Dr. Omer lives in Los Angeles, California, and specializes in emergency medicine, typically working eight-hour shifts. He works at a large tertiary care emergency department close to downtown Los Angeles. But he lives in Santa Monica. Though about 20 miles separates Dr. Omer from his workplace and his home, anyone who lives in LA—or has spent any time there—will tell you this commute is no quick trip. It can be downright protracted.

Dr. Omer's typical shifts start at random times of the day; for a 6:00 p.m. shift the commute may take up to one and a half hours.

But wait. We're getting ahead of ourselves. To make all this work, Dr. Omer must adjust his sleep schedule to have the required alertness during his shift to not make any mistakes. Once he does arrive at his hospital, he must navigate physician parking. Patients are used to scowling at all those spots reserved for doctors, grumbling all the while about how easy they've got it. Turns out the grass isn't much greener on the doctors' side. Depending on the hospital, generally it can take a doctor a good 10 to 15 minutes to find a parking spot. To make matters worse, the physician ending their shift often cannot leave until their replacement arrives, contributing to the bottleneck.

Sounds like fun, doesn't it?

Now, let's talk about the night shift. Dr. Omer usually starts this at 11:00 p.m. To accommodate his schedule, he must carefully arrange his evenings. This means if he has dinner plans with friends, he often comes wearing scrubs to leave directly for work to make it to the hospital by 10:45 p.m.

Regardless of the planning needed to ensure Dr. Omer arrives on time for his night shift, the bottom line is that while most of us are getting ready for bed—or have already gone to bed—his "day" is just starting.

As a doctor who takes his job seriously, it's mission critical to Dr. Omer that he gets to the hospital on time. He doesn't want to leave other doctors in the lurch, especially since he's been there, stuck on a shift because your replacement either shows up late or never shows.

RECKONING

We don't mention all this because we want you to feel sorry for Dr. Omer, or any other physician. Just like a firefighter or police officer who makes a conscious choice to serve their profession, he selected this career knowing what it requires, including the sacrifices.

Similarly, coauthor Chris's father chose this life. Dr. Richard Rovin has been practicing for more than three decades, specializing in neurosurgery for brain tumors. While Richard rarely missed his kids' soccer games or school performances, he did have to plan around his on-call schedule.

The Rovin family even adopted Richard's superstitions during his on-call weeks. Yes, just like a baseball player who will purposefully not change his underwear for weeks in the middle of a hot streak, Dr. Rovin falls back on little routines to keep up his luck against the dreaded work call.

Chris can still recall his family's legend about a light at the end of their driveway when they lived in Marquette, Michigan. Somehow, his dad got it into his head that if that light bulb went out while he was on call and someone fixed it, it would affect his luck. *He would be called in.*

That's why for two weeks, even in the dead of winter, he forbade anyone from changing the bulb. Emergencies in his line of work are rarely good. It's also a testament to how the waiting room experience isn't working so well—for patients *or* doctors.

MORE PAIN FROM THE FRONT LINES

Dr. Omer and Dr. Rovin's struggles with work-life balance are sadly not exceptions. They reflect the arduous obligations most every caregiver has come to expect. As *Medical News Today* reports, "Research shows that physicians work an average of 51.4 hours a week, with nearly 1 in 4 (23.5%) working 61–80 hours each week."[15] By contrast, here are the average number of hours that professionals work in some other fields:

- Management, professional, and related occupations: 42.2 hours per week
- Sales and office occupations: 41.3 hours per week
- Construction and extraction occupations: 41.5 hours per week[16]

As a helpful point of comparison, in 2023 Indeed reported these statistics concerning the number of hours lawyers work in a typical week:

- Lawyers working for large firms: 66 hours per week
- Lawyers working for small- and medium-sized firms: 42–54 hours per week
- Lawyers working for government agencies: 40 hours per week[17]

As you can see, with the exception of attorneys working for sizable organizations, doctors outpace the number of work hours for many other professions. But wait. There's more. Rockford Health System put out a comparison in 2022 breaking down work hours by specialty. A few leap out at us:

- General surgeons work an average of 60.78 hours per week.
- Internists work an average of 55 hours per week.
- Anesthesiologists work an average of 59.33 hours per week.
- Orthopedic surgeons work an average of 54.17 hours per week.
- Resident doctors work an average of 80 hours per week.[18]

Let's drill down on the last category. Resident doctors are notorious for working almost inhuman hours. As noted, the average is double the 40-hour workweek. Interestingly, *Harvard Business Review* recently asked this valid question: "Is an 80-hour workweek enough to train a doctor?" To answer this, it's worth reminding ourselves how much schooling is generally required to enter this profession. Here's the currently accepted breakdown in the United States:

- Four years of college
- Four years of medical school
- Three to ten years of residency training, depending on specialization
- Optional one to three years for a fellowship[19]

It's worth mentioning that the 80-hour workweek assigned to residents these days is 20 hours *less* than it was in the 1980s. And yet it's still grueling, leading to intense exhaustion and stress. *Harvard Business Review* reports that across several studies, more than 40 percent of U.S. physicians reported that they were burned out, and that burnout often begins in residency training.[20]

Now, to put this in more qualitative terms: Resident doctors, on average, work many more hours weekly than either Dr. Rovin or Dr. Omer, and resident doctors are stressed from such demanding time constraints. At a macro level, things have gotten so bad that George Washington University Hospital resident doctors formed a union in 2023 to combat what they view as intolerable working conditions.

Meanwhile, the physical, emotional, and psychological strain that starts when doctors are still residents continues well into their practice years. "Nearly two-thirds (63 percent) of a nationwide group of doctors and nurses said they are experiencing a moderate or great deal of burnout at work, according to a new *HealthDay*-Harris poll online survey. Those numbers jibe with figures from top medical associations." The same piece explains, "Only 57 percent of doctors say they would choose medicine as a profession again compared with 72 percent the year before."[21]

Lost in all this (needed) talk about burnout is its effect on nurses. Like doctors, they have also suffered under the strain of the waiting room experience. Consider their shifts. According to *Nurse Theory*, "Regarding the weekly schedule, nurses may work 8-hour shifts (5x) per week, 10-hour shifts (4x) per week, or 12-hour shifts (3x) per week."[22]

This is what's been generally expected. However, like doctors, nurses often put in much longer hours, especially during the COVID-19 pandemic and now, in its aftermath. World Economic Forum puts this strain in perspective, especially what's happened as a result of so many nurses not unionizing but rather leaving their profession *en masse*:

> Burnout, exhaustion and mistreatment . . . have hollowed out the world's workforce of healthcare workers.
>
> . . . The International Council of Nurses estimated that the world could be short 13 million nurses by 2030 unless action is taken to stem the tide of attrition, and bring new recruits into the healthcare workforce.[23]

It's safe to say the strain of long hours, difficult commutes, rampant staff shortages, and a host of other problems are wreaking havoc on both doctors and nurses. Way before COVID-19 strained an *already* stressed system, caregivers were inhibited from having a healthy family/dating life.

There's a reason why doctors often date only other doctors or nurses. They each understand the grueling schedules. It's a fact of life in this field.

Of course, it presents an even harder situation for women, who must juggle when to start a family (if they want to have one) with professional decisions. As Shruthi Mahalingaiah, assistant professor of environmental, reproductive, and women's health at the Harvard T. H. Chan School of Public Health's environmental health department, explains for *Boston University Today*, "Female medical students, residents, and physicians are constantly pulled in polar directions in regard to their family planning. I was a third-year OB/GYN resident when I got married and I felt that the timing for getting pregnant was not right given the stress of my work."[24]

Between the challenge of not being able to start a family or at least spend time with one's own kids, coupled with the long hours, missed events/functions, and generally a harried life, it's no wonder so many nurses are exiting. An alarming piece in *Healthcare IT News* reports that a whopping 90 percent considered leaving the profession in 2023, with 39 percent reporting anxiety, depression, and other mental health issues. Hospitals are also dealing with compounding issues because of staff shortages.[25]

To make matters worse, many nurses, like their physician counterparts, are saddled with yet another time crunch dilemma: elderly family obligations. What happens when caregivers are torn between looking after their own aging loved ones and their patients? This is a real problem. Among the so-called sandwich generation, an estimated more than 1 in 10 parents in America also must care for an aging adult.

This can require three or *more* hours a day and does not factor in their professional care obligations.

For an even deeper sense of what today's sandwich generation caregivers are up against, here are some issues contributing to burnout:

- Family strife
- Little or no personal time
- Depression and other troubling emotions

TAKEAWAY

For all these reasons and more, again, we may ask: Is it any wonder caregivers have hit their limit—much like their patients? (Just to pile on one more chilling statistic, the American Medical Association reported in 2022 that "one in five physicians say it is likely they will leave their current practice within two years. Meanwhile, about one in three doctors and other health professionals say they intend to reduce work hours in the next 12 months, according to recently published survey research."[26])

Extrapolating based on our cultural understanding of market forces, we may be inclined to think doctors and nurses will simply continue to provide the care patients have grown accustomed to. No matter all of our issues with the waiting room experience, the medical system has still provided us with top-quality care, something that makes life worth living. But as the saying goes, the only constant we can expect in life is change. It's not at all certain which part of the equation—caregivers or patients—will snap first, sowing chaos and uncertainty at an almost unimaginable level.

What *is* for certain is this unstable system cannot last. The waiting room experience has not worked well for all stakeholders for a long time. Fortunately, telemedicine promises a fix. But before we explore why it may save our system, we must learn why every day in America, too many patients are left wondering if they'll ever get the care they need to survive.

CHAPTER 3

Healthcare Deserts: Scarcity of Specialists and Care Access

Henry is a spry 89-year-old living in rural North Carolina. He's spent his whole life in the same sparsely populated county, outside of several years of military service. The man is a veritable fixture of his small community. Many consider him to be patriarch of his large extended clan. So especially as Christmas 2022 approached, Henry eagerly looked forward to a holiday gathering hosted by his grandson in a town two hours away.

What didn't he know?

Lack of access to healthcare would derail his plans—threatening his life. Days before the festivities, at a time when Henry should have felt most joyful, fear and anxiety haunted him. Henry faced a medical emergency. Considered healthy despite his advanced age, he'd been diagnosed with adult-onset epilepsy around age 40. (He had worked in forestry and learned of his epilepsy after suffering a seizure cutting down trees with a crew deep in the forest.)

Luckily, he wasn't hurt.

Still, the epilepsy changed his career. His days of wielding power equipment ended following his diagnosis back in the '70s. Even now,

Henry recalls the news—favorably. He'd reached the age where he felt sore every morning from the ongoing strain. Happily, he transitioned to a managerial position at the sawmill, a role he held until retirement. He also began a medical journey focused on maintaining quality of life living with epilepsy.

As to be expected, over the course of 50 years, Henry had experienced the ups and downs of the American medical system. His local doctor, a general practitioner and the only physician in their small town, did his best to keep up with industry changes. Also, every few years Henry would be driven by a family member to a university hospital three hours away. Here, specialists would give him a battery of tests and discuss treatment advancements. Most recently, he'd been prescribed Keppra and Depakote, medications that worked so well, Henry considered them near cures for epilepsy.

But as Henry well knew, drugs are only useful when you can take them. And he was about to experience a shortage at the worst possible time. But first, the situation Henry encountered just before Christmas is a common one in America, especially for the elderly. Henry *thought* he had an extra supply of medications, but as his current bottle dwindled to nothing, he discovered he was mistaken. Containers he believed to hold a fresh supply of his lifesaving drugs were also nearing empty.

Just days before the holiday he most cherished, Henry faced the very real possibility of an epileptic seizure that could kill him at his age. The more the medication wore off, the more he risked suffering a catastrophic injury like falling down the stairs.

Henry knew he had to act fast.

His first call was to his family doctor, the man he affectionately knew as "Dr. Pete." This physician had treated Henry's epilepsy for more than 30 years. He was also the only doctor within miles. But Henry's heart sank as he listened to Dr. Pete's voicemail. His longtime caretaker was enjoying Christmas in the Cayman Islands and wouldn't return until January. This meant medical emergencies were directed to a county hospital more than an hour away.

That didn't seem like a good option.

Henry had long mistrusted hospitals, believing most 89-year-olds entering one don't come out alive. Instead, he formulated a plan to wait for his doctor to return from vacation. He figured he could stay on the first floor of his home, avoiding dangerous situations for a week before returning to normal. Believing this to be his only option, Henry FaceTimed with his beloved grandson, the one hosting Christmas that year.

"Billy, I'm sorry," Henry began. "I'm out of my meds."

Billy was crestfallen. As the oldest living family member, Henry was the focal point of each gathering. Disappointment on the faces of Billy's wife, Sue, and son, Tyler, hurt Henry's heart, but he knew he had made the right choice.

Then Billy threw the man a curveball. "Papa, you gotta come to Christmas. Who knows how many more we'll have together?"

Sue joined in. "Billy's right. There has to be a solution."

Before Henry could argue, Henry's great-grandson Tyler spoke up. "Papa should go on the computer for his medicine."

There was a silence. Billy and Sue had used QuickMD twice for urgent care after a friend suggested telemedicine, but this was outside Henry's realm of experience. "What's that?"

"It's like FaceTime," Billy jumped in. "But you can talk to a real doctor."

Henry looked at the faces of his loved ones. He was willing to try anything if it meant seeing his grandson and all the people he so loved. Billy and Sue walked him through how to download the QuickMD app. Within 20 minutes, Henry was speaking to a physician about his situation.

The remote consultation provided Henry with a sense of ease, partly because of the comfort of being in his own home, a contrast to the usual clinical setting. The online physician, attentive to Henry's needs, promptly addressed his concerns. By the end of the appointment, a new prescription for his medications was arranged to be available at a nearby pharmacy. This timely assistance meant Henry could collect his medication before Christmas Eve, offering him peace of mind for the holidays.

Crisis averted, Henry attended the holiday celebration to great fanfare. Although his life was put in danger by a weak regional medical infrastructure, convenient telemedicine access afforded him the chance to forge lifelong memories with five generations of his beloved family.

THE NATURE VERSUS NURTURE OF YOUR PHYSICAL HEALTH

One enduring psychology debate concerns whether genetics or our environment play the larger role in our development. *Psychology Today* explains the long-running argument is to judge if an individual's characteristics and personality are more influenced by innate biological factors (the nature), or if upbringing and life experiences (the nurture) are more seminal.[1]

Most experts agree nature and nurture aren't an either-or proposition forming one's personality, a point made by cognitive psychologist Steven Pinker in a *Daedalus* article, "Why Nature and Nurture Won't Go Away."

Pinker, who teaches at Harvard, explains that nature and nurture are both, in a sense, innate and "not a set of rigid instructions for behavior." They both are equally needed in consideration of the factors that drive human behavior, "because the mind is a complex system composed of many interacting parts." To drive away one explanation in favor of the other makes no sense, especially if genetics affect behavior, he says.[2]

Despite this erudite argument, the academic debate rages on. Only it's not limited to psychology. More recently, healthcare providers have come to realize a blend of nature versus nurture occurs in our *physiological* health, not just our personality makeup.

Expanding on the concept of nature versus nurture to bodily health, we encounter a new array of variables. The nature aspect, which remains largely unchanged, includes the genetic makeup present in each cell and in our family medical histories. Advances in genetics have even enabled physicians to predict individuals' predisposition to diseases such as cancer.[3] Regarding Henry, his genetics seemingly predisposed him to robust health, as evidenced by his overall well-being approaching his 90th birthday despite his epilepsy.

Yet what may be less clear is what the nurture side of health entails. As you'd expect, nurturing our bodies often includes activities like eating a balanced diet, exercising, and drinking sufficient water. Likewise, the Centers for Disease Control and Prevention (CDC) outlines the health dangers of smoking, including cancer risks, so avoiding tobacco products is another form of nurturing our health.[4] But an entire set of variables exists about each person's life that goes far beyond what we've just described. These considerations involve who we are, where we live, even what we do for a living. Moreover, these factors can produce a dramatic health impact on every person, just as they did with Henry.

Unfortunately, every day in this country, many people like Henry have no clue how they will get their medicine. As you can imagine, it's especially dire for the unhoused who lack sufficient funds to see a doctor, much less a smartphone or Wi-Fi to connect with a physician virtually. Too often, acute problems can devolve into a life-or-death situation. This is due to *social determinants of health*, a set of living conditions and cultural factors.

THE IMPACT ON *EVERYONE*

The CDC defines *social determinants of health* (SDOH) as "the nonmedical factors that influence health outcomes. They are the conditions in which people are born, grow, work, live, and age, and the wider set of forces and systems shaping the conditions of daily life. These forces and systems include economic policies and systems, development agendas, social norms, social policies, racism, climate change, and political systems."[5]

It's important to note that SDOH don't only apply to a certain race, gender, or any other demographic or characteristic. Instead, the health of *every* American is affected positively or negatively by the SDOH they experience based on where they are born, live, learn, work, play, worship, and age. Each determinant listed here also does not exist in a vacuum.

Instead, the social determinants combine and interact with each other in complex ways. For instance, someone with poor literacy is also likely to have a low-paying job, making it harder to take time off for an annual physical. To illustrate this relationship between the SDOH and a patient's overall health, physicians at Johns Hopkins have outlined ways to integrate SDOH data into their care model.[6]

Disparate physicians, academics, and government health agencies now consider SDOH via their own subjective lenses, resulting in varying numbers of social determinants of health ranked differently by importance depending on whom you ask. Based on our experience running a leading telemedicine practice, eight SDOH are most pertinent. We review each in the following sections. You'll find that quite a few affected Henry's health journey.

SDOH 1: Generalist Proximity

In Henry's story, based on the experience of a real QuickMD patient with details changed to protect privacy, our protagonist lives in a rural area. He sees a single generalist in his hometown, with infrequent trips to a specialist, often involving considerable driving. When Henry's doctor goes on vacation, the backup option for patients needing help is a hospital hours away.

This story is not unusual.

Millions of other Americans live in so-called healthcare deserts. Lack of availability of not only specialist care but even a basic generalist is a major negative SDOH. According to GoodRx Research, more than 80 percent of U.S. counties suffer from a lack of access to services necessary to maintain good health. Data demonstrates more than 121 million Americans suffer from such paucity. That's a startling 37 percent of the population.[7]

The organization's methodology defines the myriad healthcare deserts that make up the overall statistic as places lacking pharmacies, primary care providers, hospitals, hospital beds, trauma centers, and low-cost health centers. People's "personal and financial barriers" to these things they are already missing can make it even harder for them to access needed care.[8]

Based on this data, we can see Henry's hometown is a true healthcare desert. Not enough primary care physicians serve his area—the case for more than 9 percent of U.S. counties, according to GoodRx. This means he has to drive more than 30 minutes to reach a hospital—also the reality for 20 percent of counties existing as hospital deserts. In a nod to other SDOH, GoodRx notes that lower income, limited internet access, and lack of insurance are additional barriers.[9]

But just in case you think healthcare deserts are purely a rural problem, data demolishes that myth. The *Washington Examiner* notes that these also exist in major cities, including Chicago, Los Angeles, and New York City. As GoodRx director Tori Marsh explains, "Just because you live in a very populated city doesn't necessarily mean you have the infrastructure needed. It might mean that you have fewer hospital beds; it might mean that there are not enough providers for your community."[10]

The QuickMD team considers healthcare deserts and physical proximity to care to be one of the most critical social determinants of health to tackle. By its nature, these are clear signs of inefficiencies in our legacy healthcare system. Worse yet, they are unlikely to be fixed in the near future. This creates a care gap that telemedicine can help fill, as it did in Henry's case.

SDOH 2: Employment/Income

A person's employment status and income dictate much about their lives. Some choices, based on an individual's capacity to afford things like a new car, aren't particularly linked to leading a healthy life. But once we focus specifically on healthcare spending, income becomes an important SDOH.

In 2021, CNBC reported on a survey of more than 1,000 Americans. It found 66 percent worried about affording healthcare. More than half of the most concerned also have kids, meaning they fret about care for their whole family, not just themselves. Perhaps the most eye-opening statistic is that 49 percent of respondents know they couldn't afford medical bills totaling *more than $1,000.*[11]

So how does this financial concern translate into a social health determinant? Someone working a low-level job may feel pressure not to take time off to see their doctor. They are likely to feel this strain from their employer and from their family, as time away may cause their already meager income to drop further. Put yourself in the shoes of a single mom struggling to make ends meet. How will missing half a day affect your family's ability to scrape by? Although some Americans are privileged enough to build wealth and emergency funds, the working poor are not. Only 41 percent of Americans making less than $30,000 a year can.[12]

But taking time off isn't the only problem the disadvantaged face. There is another cost involved in the hassle to see a doctor. Our single mom may have to stare down a multitude of costs and inconveniences for such a visit. Besides gas and other basic costs involved in transportation, she may need to hire a babysitter. She is also likely to have little support, such as family members who can easily pick up the kids if she is delayed. Finally, this problem can only exacerbate if she lives in a healthcare desert. That's because, like Henry, she'll have to take more time off and drive farther just to receive the kind of care residents of a wealthy suburb take for granted.

In our initial tale, income and employment affect Henry to some degree. Long since retired, he needn't worry about missing work. Yet like many seniors, Henry lives on a fixed budget. This constraint limits his ability to travel to visit specialists. It also led him to stretch out his medication, contributing to his Christmas emergency. Clearly, income and work construe an SDOH that telemedicine can support, removing many financial barriers.

SDOH 3: Education

Regardless of a person's access to care and/or their income level, maintaining health or recovering from an illness/injury can be challenging if the person struggles to understand written instructions. An inability to read materials such as medication information or a guide to physical therapy exercises can be devastating. This kind of situation transforms illiteracy from what we typically view as a societal issue into a social determinant of health.

Literacy is frequently misunderstood to be a yes-or-no question, meaning either a person can read or they cannot. Yet according to the

National Center for Education Statistics (NCES), literacy levels can be measured on a scale from 1 to 5. As recent research performed by the NCES reports, 8.1 percent of Americans are functionally illiterate. Even that doesn't tell the true story. Another 12.9 percent are level 1 readers, meaning they fail at "comparing and contrasting information, paraphrasing, or making low-level inferences." Accordingly, 21 percent—or one in five Americans—can't understand written health instructions.[13]

But the problem may be even worse.

Of those Americans who are functionally literate, 31.6 percent are at level 2, 34.6 percent are at level 3, and only 12.9 percent are at level 4 or 5. In practice, a level 2 reader and perhaps even some level 3 readers may struggle with medical instructions using unusual medical jargon. Also, illiteracy often plagues immigrants. The NCES reports that adults not born in the United States make up 34 percent of the population with low literacy skills despite making up 15 percent of the overall population.[14]

What makes education and literacy even more of an SDOH is the combination with *other* social determinants. Illiteracy hampers an individual's ability to secure a well-paying job. *Forbes* reports illiteracy costs the American economy an astounding $2.2 trillion every year.[15] Of course, Henry's relatively low education level did not restrict his ability to secure his needed medication, but he did rely on younger family members to sort through paperwork and make recommendations—a luxury many older Americans don't possess.

SDOH 4: Access to Healthy Food and Alternative Treatment

Most people recognize how the food choices we make affect our health. A juicy cheeseburger and salty fries can be a tasty treat, but if we eat them *daily*, we risk adverse health outcomes. Likewise, the Cleveland Clinic outlines a few of the health concerns related to a diet of fast food, explaining how such eating habits can raise blood pressure, drive up cholesterol levels, and lead to weight gain.[16]

But what if you live where it's hard to find something to eat that's *not* highly processed fast food? This phenomenon is called a food desert. Like the healthcare desert, when people lack nourishing options they tend to eat food that harms their health. As the United States Department of Agriculture (USDA) explains, "Even with knowledge of good nutrition and the best of intentions, some people who live in 'food desert' neighborhoods may have a difficult time accessing affordable and nutritious food because they live far from a supermarket with fresh produce and do not have easy access to transportation."[17] Similarly, the Congressional Research Service reported in 2021 that 6 percent of Americans or 19 million people live in food deserts.[18] These exist in all 50 states and the District of Columbia. When people in these areas receive instructions to eat a healthier diet, they are left with one question: *How?*

But lack of access goes beyond mainstream healthcare and food. This SDOH also considers access to alternative treatments. Some Americans find significant benefits from services like acupuncture and chiropractic care that may be unavailable to other Americans regardless of whether they live in an urban or rural area. The Harvard Health Blog reported on a new field of treating traumatic brain injury, and psychological disorders such as medication-resistant depression, with psychotropic drugs like ketamine.[19] If a person lacks access to a clinic with this novel treatment, they can't experience the potentially life-changing benefits provided by the frontiers of neuroscience.

For all the logistical might of the U.S. economy, food and health deserts are not going away. Also, alternative treatment options often stumble against the economic necessity of investing in a brick-and-mortar facility, a risk without the guarantee of a strong patient population. These factors each contribute to a serious SDOH, deeply affecting chances for a healthy life. Although telemedicine is only a partial answer to this problem, it does offer to counter such lack, thereby restoring a culture of healthy eating.

SDOH 5: Race and Cultural Issues

We purposefully omitted Henry's race from our story. Instead, we focused on his life in a healthcare desert as an illustration of how social determinants of health can affect health. Yet race and cultural issues *are* SDOH. Multiple reasons suggest that racial issues can interfere with a person's wellness. One of the primary contributors is an overall sense of poor treatment among African Americans seeking care.

A book by the Institute of Medicine, *Unequal Treatment: Confronting Racial and Ethnic Disparities in Health Care*, examines the racial divide in healthcare.[20] Of particular note, it includes findings of focus groups held within this demographic concerning attitudes about healthcare. The participants' comments are sobering—the focus group exposes rampant stereotyping by physicians, a general lack of respect by office staff, and improper diagnosis and treatment perceived to be based on race. Unsurprisingly, this produced a deep mistrust of the healthcare system.[21]

The Commonwealth Fund, focused on advancing equitable healthcare, explains a common sentiment by minorities persisting to this day:

> A growing body of researchers is exploring the factors that fuel medical mistrust, particularly among Black and other patients of color. Laura Bogart, Ph.D., a social psychologist and senior behavioral scientist at the RAND Corporation whose research has documented the effects of medical mistrust on HIV prevention and treatment outcomes, defines medical

> mistrust as an absence of trust that health care providers and organizations genuinely care for patients' interests, are honest, practice confidentiality, and have the competence to produce the best possible results.
>
> Bogart and other researchers have found that medical mistrust is not just related to past legacies of mistreatment, but also stems from people's contemporary experiences of discrimination in health care—from inequities in access to health insurance, health care facilities, and treatments to institutional practices that make it more difficult for Black Americans to obtain care.[22]

Medical mistrust among African Americans and other minorities reflects a serious negative SDOH. Yet several different mechanisms exist to counteract perceived mistrust and mistreatment that lead to poor health outcomes. One is to acknowledge that some individuals prefer doctors who look and sound like them. Researchers from Johns Hopkins who performed a study with more than 2,700 patients found that African American, Hispanic, and Asian American patients reported higher satisfaction with physicians of the same race or ethnic background. Similarly, when patients could choose their own physician, they were likelier to pick one of their own race.[23] Another study performed by researchers at Penn Medicine and published in *JAMA Network Open* found comparable results, reporting patients were inclined to give doctors the highest possible satisfaction score when they were of the same race.[24] Helpfully, by removing location barriers, telemedicine has the potential to match more Americans with a doctor with a similar ethnic and cultural background, promising better health outcomes.

Another approach to making healthcare more accessible involves integrating medical services into settings where African Americans and other minorities feel most comfortable. A notable example discussed in a 2021 episode of the *Freakonomics* podcast titled "Are Barbershops the Cutting Edge of Healthcare Delivery?" highlights a medical study. This study explored the innovative partnership between barbershops, which are pivotal community spaces. Such collaborations facilitated blood pressure screenings and on-site consultations with healthcare providers who could then connect patients with physicians for prescription medications, if necessary.

As barbershop owner Eric Muhammad explains in the podcast, barbering customers were very receptive to the program over time, because it gained their trust by showing them care. He adds that many of the men had previously seen doctors for high blood pressure, but "they weren't being serious about taking care of it. . . . They were given medication and sent home. The problem with that is there's no follow-up."[25]

Telemedicine has the ability to perform a similar follow-up. That's because digital appointments are so easy to keep. All that's required is an internet connection and electronic device. On the other hand, for certain minorities, the ability to find a doctor they feel comfortable with—and can meet on their own terms—is a winning combination for this SDOH.

SDOH 6: The Old Boys Club

In 2018, the *New York Times* published "Should You Choose a Female Doctor?" The article explores the benefits women receive when they choose to see female physicians. Edna Haber, a retired business owner, recounts choosing to see a physician because of worrying heart palpitations. Haber selected a female heart specialist based on her negative experiences with male doctors.

Author Tara Parker-Pope explains that by listening closely to Edna Haber about her "heart palpitations and feeling lightheaded," a female cardiac specialist, Dr. Goldberg, saved her life. Before that, medical tests had shown that Haber's heart was "normal," but Dr. Goldberg took Haber's concerns seriously and put her on a heart monitor for a few days. The result? A pattern that indicated Haber needed a pacemaker. "I wish all the women I know could understand how important it is to have a doctor who pays attention to them, whatever part of the body they are looking at," Haber said.[26]

Related studies demonstrate many women prefer a female obstetrician or gynecologist. One published in *Obstetrics and Gynecology* found 50.2 percent of patients favor a female OB-GYN while only 8.3 percent desired a male specialist.[27] A woman living in the wealthy suburbs of Chicago may have hundreds of such specialists to choose from, but what about a woman in Henry's town? (A lack of female physicians to suit the preferences of female patients is even more glaring when combined with the healthcare desert effect.) Like all SDOH, these factors combine to only aggravate contemporary healthcare challenges.

SDOH 7: Specialists

It's common for general practitioners and family doctors to assess and refer patients to specialists. But what happens when the specialists *aren't* available? This can be the case even when comparing two nearby geographic areas. A patient in need of an oncologist in the underprivileged community of East St. Louis, Illinois, will have dramatically less access to a needed specialist when compared to a resident of the upper-class West County area of St. Louis, Missouri, just across the Mississippi River.

Sometimes, a lack of specialists can reach crisis levels, not only in a particular town or county but for an entire state. The *Albuquerque Journal* reported in February 2023 on this issue. One interviewed patient had been waiting six months to be seen about a potentially cancerous golf-ball-sized mass in her intestines.[28] This example perfectly shows how a lack of specialists is a negative SDOH.

According to the *Journal*, many factors contribute to a shortage of specialists, including high medical malpractice premiums and having to pay gross receipts taxes on medical services provided. No matter the reasons driving the shortage, the numbers are startling to anyone who cares about the health and wellness of New Mexico residents:

> New Mexico in 2021 had 1,649 primary care physicians, 700 less than the state had in 2017, according to the New Mexico Health Care Workforce Annual Report. The state is 334 primary care physicians below national provider-to-population benchmarks, according to the report.

In addition, more than 60 OB-GYNs had left the state, and there was a huge lack of psychiatrists. Compounding the problem, "the average age of a physician in New Mexico is older than 50," meaning that the shortages will continue as doctors retire.[29]

As you'll recall, a lack of specialists played a role in Henry's story. The nearest epileptologist (a neurologist focusing on epilepsy treatment) resided nearly two hours away from Henry's home. Yes, Henry saw a specialist every few years, but not as often as his primary care physician would prefer. Thankfully, as in this case, telemedicine *already* demonstrates a strong ability to break down walls between patients and specialists—same as for general practitioners.

SDOH 8: Transportation

Even when someone has healthcare options available, there is *still* a giant bridge to cross: getting to one's appointment. Elderly patients like Henry often are not able to drive long distances to see a doctor. According to the American Public Transportation Association, 45 percent of Americans lack access to public transportation, so that isn't an option either.[30]

In fact, 3.6 million Americans fail to obtain the medical care needed because they struggle to reach a doctor's office or hospital, according to research by the American Hospital Association (AHA).[31] Imagine the struggle of underprivileged and older patients expected to travel to a different region or to board an airplane to another state (or even another country) to get care. Transportation is an SDOH with serious consequences. It's also a social determinant that can be immediately eliminated through telemedicine because the doctor's office visit is virtual.

WHEN THERE'S ONLY ONE SPECIALIST IN TOWN

Author Chris Rovin witnessed SDOH in action growing up in Michigan's remote Upper Peninsula, known as the "UP" by Midwesterners. His father, Dr. Richard Rovin, was the only neurological surgeon taking call in the Upper Peninsula for years in the early 1990s. Chris watched how difficult it was for his dad to step away and take vacations, knowing patients had nowhere else to turn.

In the past, physicians sometimes turned to temporary locum tenens staff. These temporary stand-in staffers "hold the place of" the physician (a literal translation of the Latin phrase) when the physician travels. Locum tenens positions were expensive and difficult to fulfill, especially for specialists like Dr. Rovin. Locum tenens systems still exist today in remote areas such as Native American reservations and rural nursing services, as well as in underserved urban areas. Knowing their benefits, we believe telemedicine can re-create—and even reimagine—the locum tenens system to take the burden off local doctors and the healthcare system itself.

Still, like all aspects of telemedicine, this plan works best when it artfully weaves together the advantages of telehealth and legacy healthcare providers—what we witnessed concerning Henry. But before we can explore telemedicine's true potential, we must journey back in time a bit, again. It's time to examine America's recent history, illustrating why this country took so long to embrace its many advantages. Especially why it took so long to help people like our long-suffering epileptic patient.

CHAPTER 4

The Internet Ate ~~the World~~ Medicine

As Mary approached her 70th birthday in 2018, she reflected proudly on roles she'd played in her large (and growing) family. Mary was a mother and grandmother, but not only that—she was also more tech savvy than her children. It amused her grandchildren endlessly how their parents usually called Grandma for tech help instead of the other way around. Mary's oldest grandchild even took to calling her a "leet," gamer slang for *elite*. (Mary knew just what he meant because she understood internet culture.)

The reason Mary spent so much time and energy keeping up with tech came back to memories of her *own* grandmother, Mildred. She recalled Mildred as a loving figure, but one who was completely tech illiterate. That probably isn't a strong enough term. Mary's grandmother was technophobic. As Mary recalls, Grandma Mildred was not in favor of microwave ovens because of the radiation she believed they gave off. She wouldn't allow one in her kitchen. Mary remembers complaining how she couldn't even "nuke" her fish sticks. As Grandma Mildred would say, "When your friends are infertile, they'll wish they waited for the oven, deary."

But Mildred's distaste for tech extended beyond food preparation. Long after most families owned a color TV, she kept her small black-and-white set. Whenever she was asked about it, she'd say, "This one suits me just fine." Her ancient relic lasted well into the '70s, at which point Mary bought her a new color model. Mildred's response? "*That's* the color of Jimmy Stewart's hair?"

Mildred didn't embrace technology until the end of her life. That's when she became a devoted viewer of the Home Shopping Network, a pleasure for seniors hunting for a deal long before the web gave us eBay and Amazon. Her attitude influenced Mary's life in other big ways. As much as she loved Grandma Mildred, Mary knew she would be a *different* kind of grandmother.

For one thing, she recognized her grandmother's Luddite attitude often left Mildred at a disadvantage. As technology became a bigger part of society, Mary worked to stay on top of it. When raising her own kids, this meant mastering phone trees and fax machines. A generation later, she knew she had to become an internet whiz to keep her family protected.

Safety for her children and grandchildren had always been of special importance to Mary. She even considered her technical know-how to be a way to contribute to the ongoing care of the next generation. In 2016, this gambit paid off big time. One of her grandchildren, Cody, then 13, was active on social media. Mary followed the teen's account on Twitter before he joined Discord, a platform popular with gamers to organize play sessions and voice chat during matches. Making it a habit to keep an eye on the activities of her kids, she noticed something disturbing going on with her young grandson.

But first, it should be acknowledged that Cody's posts were not out of the ordinary. Mostly clips from *Fortnite*, gaming memes, and cute animal videos, his content was innocuous. What troubled Mary was *who* interacted with his posts. Along with accounts clearly belonging to friends, almost everything the boy made was favorited and replied to by an account of a 28-year-old male one state away. Logging into Discord one day, Mary discovered the man also had an account in the same chat group as her grandson. To Mary, this looked odd—and she wasted no time getting it all straightened out.

Mary appealed to her daughter. "Find out from Cody who this man is."

The boy said he thought he was just another gamer. "But he does creep me out. Especially 'cause of how often he DMs [direct messages] me."

The family immediately blocked the stranger on all platforms. Next, Cody's parents wrote to him, threatening to report him to the police if he contacted their boy again. Mary also worked with Cody to set ground rules so the same thing wouldn't happen again. Though scary at the time, Mary continued to consider technology a clear positive in her life.

Actually, innovation brought Mary's family closer together, enriching their life experiences. She often used FaceTime to video chat with her son and grandson across the country. When she was young, she hardly ever saw a cousin who lived an hour away. But smartphones can bridge much farther gaps than that. Besides using FaceTime and becoming a social media expert, Mary learned Italian using Duolingo, and gave back to her community by teaching computer literacy classes to other seniors at her local library.

To be sure, tech enhanced nearly every part of her life—with one glaring exception. Back in 2018, Mary found herself wondering why she could do almost anything on the internet *except* talk to her doctor and/or manage her health. This thought often struck her while gardening. She could order all the home improvement supplies she needed from Amazon and other vendors—including live ladybugs to eat pests; she could even connect via video chat with a botanist to diagnose issues with her plants to improve her harvest. So why couldn't she take care of her own health the same way?

As it turns out, healthcare back then was more of a hassle for Mary than ever. She regularly saw two doctors. One, her trusted family caregiver, had moved to the far suburbs, creating an hour drive each way—fighting against traffic. Mary had to cancel more than one appointment because of trouble commuting. Visiting the other doctor she trusted was even harder to manage. Mary had been seeing a rheumatologist who provided her excellent arthritis care. Unfortunately, he moved across the state line because of unfavorable regulations and skyrocketing malpractice costs. In fact, so many specialists had left for the same reason that Mary didn't know if she could find a replacement.

Again, questions swirled around in her head constantly. "If we have the technology available to make video conference calls and the logistics set up to ship anything to anywhere, why am I stuck driving for hours, searching for a doctor to see me in his office?" Finally, during the COVID-19 pandemic, when both of Mary's providers began offering telemedicine, a new question emerged: "Why'd this take so long?"

This was a mystery to far more people than just Mary. But it is a question without a simple answer. Instead, the disconnect between the power of the internet and the delivery of healthcare is one with many contributing factors. Let's explore them now.

HOW THE INTERNET BECAME PART OF EVERYDAY LIFE

Mary, like most seniors, worked most of her career without computers. This is hard to imagine for younger professionals today who rely on computers, smartphones, and the web for practically every part of their job. The Computer History Museum notes that Apple released the original Macintosh computer in 1984, the first PC she used in an office setting.[1] Around that time, Mary's kids were learning about computers on Apple machines Steve Jobs flooded school systems with, brilliantly creating a market by exposing as many schoolchildren to his products as possible.[2] But while she used a computer at work and the kids played *Oregon Trail* at school, the internet as we know it didn't yet exist. Also, online connectivity was a complex process and the exclusive province of techies willing to learn arcane login processes for bulletin board systems (BBSs) and other rudimentary online forums.

Although no one knew what a "dot com" was back then, many people were suddenly using computers daily. This set up the rapid advancement of the internet in three waves. It is useful to understand the trio to add context to telemedicine's development as QuickMD practices it in 2024.

Internet 1.0: AOL and Online Dating

Mary's first experiences with the internet would be hardly recognizable to Generation Z. Her family, like millions of others, dutifully bought a home computer from Gateway, plugged their 56K modem into a phone jack, and installed AOL from a CD they got free in the mail. (Tech site Vox calls AOL's iconic CDs "history's greatest junk mail," noting the company sent out an estimated *one billion* between 1993 and 2006. AOL used a bold marketing ploy to jump-start what would soon become known as the internet, and it worked.[3])

Like many families, Mary's family initially used AOL for its rudimentary chat features. They were also introduced to email by the service. The *Washington Post* reports that by 1997, AOL had more than 19,000 chat rooms. Users spent more than 1 million hours chatting per day.[4] Those aren't big numbers compared to YouTube and Facebook, especially not these days, but when compared to the pioneering online services preceding AOL, the usage was *astronomical.*

By 1998, the online lifestyle went mainstream. In "The History of Online Dating: A Timeline from Paper Ads to Websites," author Hayley Matthews explains this is the year the smash hit movie *You've Got Mail*, starring Tom Hanks and Meg Ryan, came out.[5] Named after the iconic AOL email sound clip, the movie normalized the online dating concept.

Although no one in Mary's family found love online, a close friend met her future husband on Match.com, which launched in 1995.[6] Dating sites were just *one* of the services popping up as the internet ballooned from walled gardens like AOL to the World Wide Web. Mary and her clan soon became familiar with hearing web addresses included in ads. Her husband even bought a copy of the *Internet Yellow Pages*, a (now antiquated) guide to websites in paper form.[7] She still loves telling her grandkids about it, and recalls the oldest asking, "Why didn't you just google it?"

His jaw hit the floor when she told him Google didn't yet exist. During this era, from the early 1990s to the early 2000s, the internet expanded rapidly. Yahoo! was the top search engine, and Wall Street pushed vast sums into the dot-com bubble, only to see it burst in short order.[8] Even so, the web was here to stay. It wasn't yet an indispensable part of daily life, but the writing was on the wall.

Internet 2.0: How Many Likes Did Your Post Get?

By the early 2000s, Mary's kids were entering a workforce where the internet was no longer a novelty, but rather, a daily tool. She remembers an incident from 2004 where her husband handed her son Tyler a copy of the newspaper want ads. "Son," he began. "I don't see you trying to find a job. Let's go through this to see who's hiring."

Tyler looked at him like he'd just sprouted a second head. "Um, Dad, the paper is how *you* found a job breaking rocks back in the Stone Age."

Mary had to stifle a laugh before cutting in. "Tyler's got a point, honey.

Job searches are online nowadays." Later, their boy would amaze his parents by showing off his profile on newly launched LinkedIn, billed as a social media platform for professionals.[9] Investigating the new service, Mary read an interview with LinkedIn cofounder Konstantin Guericke, reflecting that his words contained wisdom on how the internet could have a future positive impact.[10]

LinkedIn wasn't the only social media platform, of course. All of Mary's children had accounts on MySpace, which the *New York Times* described as the "king of social networks" in social media's early days.[11] Still, Mary's spidey sense was triggered by the concept of strangers "liking" and "following" posts from her children, especially her daughter. However, she knew her kids were smart and trusted them to keep their online friend group to those in their actual social circle.

Yet as Facebook and other modern social media took off, this would all change. Before long, people were meeting others with similar interests all around the country, even the world. Online friendships and relationships weren't new, but "netizens" got to know each other better than ever thanks to social media profiles and a wide range of consumer-friendly chat apps.

The boom in broadband internet supported much of this development. Pew Research reports that only 1 percent of American adults had access to broadband internet in early 2000. By early 2004, that figure had jumped to 25 percent. By 2006, 42 percent were on the internet with a high-speed connection.[12] The sudden availability of massive bandwidth meant video flooded the typical consumer's screen from YouTube and on social media. Two-way video calls were now feasible too, with Skype being the most popular app.[13] Though Mary was well on her way to being a technology whiz, she couldn't have predicted the internet would make the leap from her desk to her pocket, along with the pockets of practically everyone worldwide.

Internet 3.0: Living by the Glow of Your Screen

According to a *Business Insider* retrospective on the Apple iPhone, Steve Jobs's first smartphone, released in 2007, is a "primitive brick."[14] But at the time, it changed the world, bringing the power of the internet everywhere we went. Suddenly social media posts featured pictures from events, and we were all living a form of "mediated reality," experiencing and interacting with the world via screens and technology.[15]

People were now connected to the internet and to each other at all times. It wasn't long before Mary got her first FaceTime video call from her grandson moments after he hit a home run in a Little League game. She may have been hundreds of miles away at the time, but she soaked in the joy of his triumph through the power of tech—and her family's data plan.

In our modern internet era, how we work and play has radically changed, thanks to being always online. Mary's son works for a major corporation. For years, he's used his iPhone to manage a national team via the workplace organization app Slack.[16] He leveraged Zoom videoconferencing years before the COVID-19 pandemic struck. Mary's extended family members have also long used apps like Tinder and Bumble, making the online dating in *You've Got Mail* seem quaint by comparison.

Nowadays, the typical person spends much of their day with screens and technology. We use smartphones, tablets, and laptops to stay in touch with family and friends, conduct business, learn new skills, watch films and shows, listen to music, and of course, to shop. According to Mary, her grandkids would have trouble completing *any* of these tasks without a smartphone.

Such an utter acceptance of mediated reality did not come without costs. Mary felt deep concern about her grandchildren's safety on social media now that they had embraced the habit of oversharing personal info and capturing every moment of their lives with their phones. Beyond the incident where she once protected her grandson, Mary also spotted troubling mental health issues in a granddaughter who became a heavy Instagram user.

It turns out Facebook's leadership also knew what dangers teen girls faced on the company's platform, a fact exposed by the *Wall Street Journal*'s "Facebook Files" series published in 2021. The *Journal* reported that the constant comparison game young women engage in on social media, including Facebook and Instagram, can damage their body image.[17]

For all the ups and downs of mediated reality and now the smartphone age, one thing is clear. America had the tech and consumer savvy in place for telemedicine to succeed *long* before the pandemic sprang to life. Yet Mary's question before her 70th birthday still stands: Why wasn't she attending telemedicine appointments in 2018 as she would a few short years later? One contributing factor is a deep distrust of how Silicon Valley does business.

THE CLASH OF INNOVATION AND HEALTHCARE VALUES

The tech world has long operated under a particular ethos. It prizes innovation and profitability over any other factor. Perhaps Mark Zuckerberg offers the best distillation of this philosophy in a letter to prospective shareholders back in 2012. As explained by *Wired*, the Facebook CEO said, "We have a saying: 'Move fast and break things.' The idea is that if you never break anything, you're probably not moving fast enough."[18]

Of course, the worship of innovation goes far beyond one company. It's baked into the DNA of practically every tech organization. Sometimes Silicon Valley's idea of "breaking things" means breaking laws, or at least bending them. One such example is Uber. The ride-sharing giant has engaged in efforts around the world to innovate—while crushing competition. As reported by the *Guardian*, the American-based company secretly paid France's Emmanuel Macron to lobby in their favor against his own nation's taxi industry back when he was minister of the economy. When this arrangement was exposed through leaks, Aurélien Taché, a French parliament member, said, "It's almost like a bad thriller—meetings and rendezvous that were hidden," adding that "it's a state scandal."[19]

Uber's innovation also turned more sinister as it focused on combating rival ride-share companies. *Fortune* reported in 2017 that the company ran a clandestine program code-named "Hell" (of all things) to track drivers for rival Lyft's service. Uber then leveraged this data to inform all sorts of tactical decisions aimed at squeezing out its competitor.[20]

Now, put yourself in Mary's shoes. Would you want companies like Uber accessing all of your health data in a "Hell" program devised to put rival doctors out of business? Actually, you don't need to be a 70-year-old tech whiz to fear this outcome. Anyone would.

But an emphasis on speed to innovation hasn't only led many Silicon Valley organizations to break laws or develop underhanded business practices. It's also produced negative impacts on humanity in a manner much more closely related to the healthcare industry—like sending driverless car crash victims to the hospital.

Elon Musk's Tesla, Google's Waymo, and even Uber have rushed driverless car tech to market when it wasn't ready for prime time. CNN reported in 2020 that an Uber driverless car hit and killed a pedestrian as the "safety driver" was looking at their smartphone.[21] Tesla, the largest electric vehicle company, has apparently applied Zuckerberg's "move fast and break things"[22] ethos to cars, and by extension, human bones: Tesla drivers are "involved in more accidents than drivers of any other brand."[23]

Inside EVs, a site dedicated to covering electric cars and by no means a critic of Musk's company, notes the National Highway Transportation Safety Administration (NHTSA) currently has an astonishing 41 open investigations of Tesla's full-self-driving tech concerning accidents.[24] Again, Silicon Valley flunks "the Mary test." No one who knows how companies rushed half-baked "self-driving" cars to market may want to hand over medicine to reckless innovators without real assurances. After all, they could develop surgery robots just as likely to amputate the wrong limb as they are to help you heal.

A second factor contributing to mistrust of tech in healthcare is how the internet giants became leviathans in the first place—profitability. A new breed of internet Goliaths like Google, Facebook, and Snapchat learned the lessons of the dot-com bubble, focusing not only on cool products but on their monetization. In the case of the biggest, most successful exemplars, this business model is based on vacuuming up every personal detail of users' lives.

Harvard professor Shoshana Zuboff coined the term "surveillance capitalism" to describe this phenomenon. She revealed Zuckerberg and other Silicon Valley players wrested control of the web by making *people* the products, earning astronomical returns in the process. Zuboff published *The Age of Surveillance Capitalism* in 2019 to document the troubling way Silicon Valley turns personal details into huge profits.[25]

As the *Guardian* reports, Zuboff's book details the problems with "the new economic order" of big tech and data gathering, led by megacorporations such as Google and Facebook. It explains how the personal information these companies gather has been used not only to predict our behavior but also to influence it and how this negatively affects democracy and freedom.[26]

Americans are often reminded of the surveillance capitalism model when it pops up in real life. How many times have you seen an ad on your phone or computer related to something you just mentioned to a friend or family member? Tech companies swear they aren't listening, but it's hard to reconcile such declarations with troubling facts.

Such a mixed backdrop has led to a revolt against healthcare data entering the surveillance capitalism system. Or at least it's produced valid concerns about it. *Becker's Hospital Review* reports there are currently 18 hospitals and health systems facing lawsuits for sharing patient data with Facebook and Google.[27] Many of these websites allege hospitals sent protected health info to tech giants based on tracking tech. It's clear from both these lawsuits and the general climate of America's uneasy relationship with Silicon Valley that most of us don't want surveillance capitalists to have *any* of our health data, let alone doctors' notes and the results of our most private medical exams. Yet barriers to bringing tech to healthcare extend beyond cultural norms and into the world of government regulation.

RYAN HAIGHT AND TELEMEDICINE'S LONG DARK WINTER

The opioid epidemic is one of America's greatest healthcare challenges. Before overdoses started piling up, the FDA approved OxyContin in 1995, the opioid most intimately related to the crisis we've suffered for many years now. Purdue Pharma, owned by the Sackler family, once marketed OxyContin as safe and nonaddictive. But as a paper by Art Van Zee published in the *American Journal of Public Health* notes, Purdue Pharma promoted "more liberal use of opioids," and sustained-release opioids in particular, to primary care doctors, who began to prescribe more OxyContin. By 2003, "nearly half of all physicians prescribing OxyContin were primary care physicians." This caused concern among some experts that that "primary care physicians were not sufficiently trained in pain management or addiction issues" and, because of time constraints, were not allowing enough "time for evaluation and follow-up of patients with complicated chronic pain."[28]

Purdue would later file for Chapter 11 bankruptcy, and the Sackler family was forced to pay out $4.5 billion to settle claims over the drug nicknamed "hillbilly heroin."[29] Of course, this means little to so many grieving families who have lost (and continue to lose) loved ones to the opioid crisis. Worse, much of the public maintains a stereotypical image of such victims. They are perceived to be strung-out addicts in big cities or backward country folk popping "Oxy" in rural areas. Only opioid abuse doesn't care about race, education, socioeconomic status, or any other factor. Far too often, its victims look like Ryan Haight.

The *Washington Post* once described Ryan as a "teenager smitten with Quiksilver sports clothes, baseball cards, and downloading music. He was an honor student, a tennis player, a clerk at a discount store and just barely 18."[30] More importantly, his parents seemed to be doing everything right. His surgeon father and nurse mother kept the family computer in a public space to monitor his internet usage. Unfortunately, the debit card they gave him to buy baseball cards through eBay was being used for a darker purpose.

Ryan had fallen into a spiral of drug experimentation and addiction, sending fake prescriptions to pharmacies in other states and foreign countries. These allowed him to receive drugs in the mail, including Vicodin. He died of a Vicodin overdose on February 12, 2001. One pharmacist who filled Ryan's prescriptions was later brought up on federal charges that sent him to prison.[31] But the teen's death had far more serious consequences on telemedicine's future. His unfortunate passing exposed weak regulations for online prescription drug sales, making it easy for Ryan and others to access scheduled drugs.

The tragic incident ultimately led to the Ryan Haight Online Pharmacy Consumer Protection Act, passed in 2008. The Haight Act, as it's popularly known, brought new restrictions to the intersection of medicine and the web. Internet pharmacies could no longer operate in a "Wild West" environment under the law. Instead, they had to follow rigorous standards. Likewise, telemedicine practitioners were further required to see patients in person periodically to prescribe controlled substances to them.

Unfortunately, such (well-intentioned) restrictions defeat the purpose of telehealth for patients and doctors alike in many cases. Or at least hinder them. The Haight Act established strong regulations to a nascent telemedicine industry not unlike the Dark Web. Before the Haight Act, patients could complete a questionnaire to get a painkiller prescription *without ever speaking to a doctor*. These scripts were then shopped around to third-party pharmacies like the one that supplied Ryan Haight with the Vicodin leading to his death.

One of the most infamous "online pill mill" practitioners was Paul le Roux, an encryption and programming expert and Zimbabwean national. Paul le Roux was convicted and is now serving 25 years in United States federal prison for running the pirate pharmacy network RX Limited, generating "hundreds of millions of euros in revenue annually" by selling opioids.[32]

The actions of people like le Roux have had a twisted silver lining worldwide. Their actions demonstrated pent-up demand among patients for telehealth services. People like Mary had long wished for the convenience and ease of seeing their doctors online—after all, this is where so much of daily life now takes place. They also wanted to have their prescriptions filled by mail. But those needs weren't being met, especially not after the Haight Act. The situation around telemedicine in the United States wouldn't shift until COVID-19 transformed nearly everything in our culture—seemingly overnight.

HOW TELEMEDICINE CHANGED—AND MAY KEEP CHANGING—HEALTHCARE

Many professionals, sometimes called "the laptop class," seamlessly transitioned to remote work during the COVID-19 lockdown. Thanks to our familiarity with mediated reality, coordinating work via helpful productivity tools and Zoom meetings was easy. The fact that many people could "go to their jobs" in pajamas was like icing on the cake.

But the medical transition looked—and still looks—quite different.

The event that most affected telemedicine—resulting in QuickMD's rapid growth and the book you're reading—was the declaration of a public health emergency in 2020.[33] This had several immediate impacts on the Haight Act. It rolled back requirements for in-person visits to prescribe controlled substances, along with removing secondary U.S. Drug Enforcement Administration (DEA) registrations. It gave the states power to bypass certain medical licensing and prescription laws. The emergency also instructed Medicare to pay for telemedicine appointments the same way it compensates for in-person visits. Perhaps most importantly, it sent a message to medical practitioners: telemedicine is at last emerging from the shadows.

When the government demonstrated that it was taking telemedicine seriously, both doctors and pharmacists could see that remote care was no longer a niche service to be ignored. It was finally time for healthcare to catch up to tech—like Mary had desired all along. This process spurred the growth of QuickMD and immediate patient acceptance of the care they could receive via a video call. In short, visiting a doctor was now as easy as joining Zoom for work, and typically less painful. The question now on the minds of the public was: Will regulators and politicians at state and federal levels enable telemedicine to continue to make America healthier?

It's our sincere hope the answer is yes. Already, telemedicine has proven to be a major contributor to the fight against opioid overdoses during the COVID-19 lockdown, especially through QuickMD's combination of telemedicine and medication-assisted treatment (MAT) for addiction. This is TeleMAT, based on the medication Suboxone (a combination of the drugs buprenorphine and naloxone). According to the federal government, 40 percent of America's counties lack a doctor that can prescribe MAT.[34] Particularly, African Americans fighting opioid use disorder (OUD), also known as MOUD,[35] are most at risk for not having a caregiver to effectively treat their addiction with these lifesaving drugs.[36] Telemedicine's ability to act as the solution to this problem is jeopardized if vital provisions related to the Haight Act are not extended—which is exactly what proposed legislation aims to do.

Thankfully, all hope is not lost. The Telehealth Response for E-prescribing Addiction Therapy Services Act (TREATS), introduced by then-senator Rob Portman (R-OH) and Senator Sheldon Whitehouse (D-RI), seeks to permanently expand telemedicine resources to treat opioid addiction.[37] The TREATS Act will enable TeleMAT to continue helping patients without having to worry that its legal underpinning could be yanked at any moment.

Portman urges that the proposed rule be made federal law. As he says, "Throughout the pandemic, this telehealth flexibility has saved lives. . . . This proposed rule seeks to increase access by reducing barriers for both treatment providers and patients needing treatment for opioid addiction."[38]

What's more, Portman has championed telemedicine in other ways, including the Comprehensive Addiction and Recovery Act (CARA). CARA 3.0, which is currently under consideration, includes almost $800 million in funding for addiction recovery.[39] It also recognizes that along with stopping the flow of dangerous drugs like fentanyl, we must help addicts overcome the all-consuming need for these drugs. Crucially, CARA includes funding for TeleMAT as long as the provider is in the same state as their patient. It also permanently allows providers to prescribe MAT drugs, including buprenorphine, without requiring an in-person visit.

Undeniably, the COVID-19 pandemic was the catalyst that brought telemedicine mainstream for patients like Mary who had long hoped for a technological solution to a pressing need—medicine. But it was an excellent experience for both doctors and patients, particularly those suffering from opioid addiction, that will power remote care into the future. That won't be possible based solely on a stopgap measure to address a health emergency. Instead, among other things, it requires visionary lawmakers like Rob Portman and others who recognize telemedicine's power to produce positive health outcomes.

In Part II, we dive into why telemedicine holds the key to the medical crisis, one that's been exacerbated by deepening cracks in our brick-and-mortar healthcare foundation.

PART II

TODAY

CHAPTER 5

Why Telemedicine Will Solve Today's Medical Crisis

We start the last few chapters with stories inspired by real-life QuickMD patients. This chapter's tale is slightly different—it's still based on the true experiences of a telemedicine patient, but without the successful application of QuickMD's technology, you wouldn't be reading this book in its present form. This is the story of coauthor Michael Ashley turning to telehealth to help his young son, whom we'll call Justin.

Prior to our story, Michael lived and worked in Southern California for most of his adult life. He built a dual career working in both Hollywood and publishing, but especially after the birth of his two children, the feast-or-famine Tinseltown economy became less attractive. As Michael's focus shifted, he realized SoCal might not be the best place for his young family. High costs, increasing crime, and the lack of green space all contributed to a growing desire to get out of the big city—to (literally) seek greener pastures.

The Ashleys moved from Orange County to rural Idaho in late 2020. Their new home was a big hit for the whole family. Michael had a roomy study to run his writing business. His wife liked experiencing all four seasons, and their kids now had an incredible amount of space to play in. They all enjoyed a slower, relaxed pace of being, as well as access to wildlife and forests. Actually, it was their proximity to so much new plant life that caused them problems.

Shortly after moving, Michael's young son Justin began showing concerning symptoms. He was sneezing more than usual and seemed to have a perpetual runny nose and watery eyes. Michael and his wife wondered if he'd caught a cold or even had COVID-19. His symptoms weren't severe, so his parents didn't panic. Noting Justin didn't have a fever, they decided to monitor how he felt for a few days before acting.

Unfortunately, Justin's symptoms didn't improve. Even though their four-year-old wasn't a complainer, it was clear he was suffering. He sniffled throughout the day and would constantly need someone to wipe his runny nose. Before long, he also developed an itchy rash. Believing Justin was dealing with allergies to plants and/or airborne allergens, they decided to take him to the doctor, having no idea they were about to enter a broken health system that's devolved into a labyrinth of frustration.

Michael and his wife hadn't spent much time contemplating medical care in Idaho before their move. The reason is simple—the Ashley family is young, and all four members had been graced with good health. Their focus was more on schools, childcare, and economic opportunity, largely the emphasis of most Americans. Therefore, it isn't all that surprising they were caught off guard by how hard it would be to get help for their son.

The Ashleys found a caring pediatrician in a nearby town. Both children received annual checkups from her, allowing their parents to form a relationship with the doctor. That pediatrician was their first call when they realized Justin had allergies. She recommended their son see a specialist. Michael recalls thinking, "No problem. Let's pull up allergists in our zip code."

What he found floored him—Michael had no idea they had moved into a *specialist desert*. Still thinking like a resident of an upper-middle-class SoCal neighborhood, Michael expected to find multiple nearby specialists in allergy treatment, including pediatric allergists. Instead, he located *none* in his area. The closest allergist who would even take kids as patients had an office more than 60 minutes away in Washington, just outside of Spokane.

Michael's wife ran the search again, thinking something had to be off. All the while, Michael fumed. "We live in America. Aren't there supposed to be doctors *everywhere*?" Still, Michael had no clue as to the full extent of the problem. He couldn't imagine all the frustrating hoops they'd be expected to jump through just to get their son the care big-city residents take for granted.

Next, Michael's wife contacted their insurance carrier to learn more about their coverage. She was told they must first take Justin to a pediatrician in Spokane just to write a referral to an allergist in the same state. Then they would be at the mercy of that busy doctor's schedule to determine when Justin could achieve any relief from his allergies—which had only worsened as the family got deeper into their first Idaho spring.

At this point, Michael began contemplating all the time and cost involved in helping his son. And others like him. Besides the major traveling involved and the high price of gas it entailed—especially in an inflationary economy—Michael and his wife would have to take time off for appointments. This was especially tough for young professionals like them. Every parent knows it's difficult to concentrate in a waiting room full of sick and crying kids, let alone conduct Zoom calls or make edits to a book like the very one you're reading!

Of course, Michael and his wife also weren't thrilled with the idea of exposing their son to further medical complications by taking him to a doctor's office filled with ill children. Considering the logistical nightmare that the legacy healthcare system placed before their family, Michael's wife implored him, "Can't you find a better way to get Justin in front of a doctor? I can't stand to see him suffering."

Armed with new resolve, Michael made some calls. More than one colleague offered the same answer: "Go the telemedicine route." Taking the baton from Michael, his wife went further. She devoted herself to a crash course on telemedicine, discovering that Justin could see a pediatrician from the comfort of home to satisfy the insurance company and then meet with a highly qualified pediatric allergist—also from home. The allergist was more than a five-hour drive from the Ashleys' new place, yet had immediate openings, thanks to telemedicine's efficiency.

Michael recalls thinking this all sounded too good to be true. His family's experience with telemedicine proved otherwise. Sidestepping logistical nightmares—plus the legacy healthcare system's ever-skyrocketing costs—Justin did see a pediatric specialist just days after initial contact. The allergist reviewed his symptoms and medical history, ordering a test to be performed by a lab just 30 minutes from the Ashleys' home. Testing was far simpler than at a doctor's office. The family simply walked in at the appointed time and a qualified technician performed it. As soon as the results came back, determining the allergy's culprit—juniper pollen—the allergist prescribed an appropriate medication. Justin bounced back, good as new.

This whole experience shocked Michael and his wife.

They had no idea how hard it would be to see an allergist in 2023. Fortunately, their child regained his health (and his love of the woods) far faster and at far cheaper cost than anticipated after learning they lived in a specialist desert. Justin was also able to be seen by a qualified pediatric allergist. Furthermore, Michael knew he'd just personally experienced the future of medicine, especially since the QuickMD team's founders had been instrumental in leading him to their son's caregiver. Most pertinent to our discussion, before his family ever enjoyed telemedicine's successful application, Michael suffered through the same crisis presently roiling our legacy healthcare system.

Extrapolating from this personal experience, we'll now explore many of the systemic challenges plaguing America's traditional care model. Unfortunately, as Michael's (recent) story shows, these problems are only exacerbating with each passing day. Yet telemedicine promises to turn this dire situation around. Just like it did for the Ashleys.

AN EXPERT'S VIEW ON OUR DEEPENING CRISIS

Michael may have just awoken to the healthcare nightmare plaguing our nation, but it isn't news to his coauthors. Chris Rovin, Jared Sheehan, and Dr. Talib Omer all possess firsthand experiences with the systemic challenges threatening our citizens' quality of life. These issues led them to launch QuickMD as a remedy to much of what Michael went through with his son.

Beyond receiving QuickMD's unique perspective, there is great value in gaining insights as large and complex as the legacy healthcare system itself. For this expertise we tapped industry expert Randall Hallett. For years, he's been pushing up against healthcare's woes, but in an utterly different way.

Hallett built a sterling reputation as a fundraising practitioner, including as the chief development officer (CDO) of the University of Nebraska Medical Center. Fundraising is an especially major component of effective healthcare delivery, since the American Hospital Association reports roughly 57 percent of community hospitals are nonprofits.[1] Hallett later assumed the presidency of a leading nonprofit consultancy, where he worked closely with major health systems, universities, and social service agencies to enhance their fundraising capabilities. Today, as the CEO and founder of Hallett Philanthropy, he continues to empower healthcare nonprofits, helping them to reach their ambitious fundraising targets.

As the coauthor of the 2023 book *Vibrant Vulnerability*[2] with Michael Ashley, Hallett has assumed a leadership role in navigating America's healthcare crisis. Hallett believes the solution to our puzzle requires fitting together disparate pieces, one of which is telemedicine. He also recognizes the importance of documenting root causes to understand how we got here. As Hallett explains, "One of my favorite sayings I share with clients involves a bit of old Gaelic wisdom: 'Some people make things happen, others watch things happen. Then there are those who wonder what just happened.' Well, in healthcare, we have many people wondering what the heck *did* just happen."[3]

What Got Us into This Mess

While many factors have contributed to our current crisis, one of the most fundamental antecedents is the terrible economic position most hospitals now find themselves in. As Hallett explains, "Hospitals generally negotiate contracts for services to patients on both a short- and long-term basis. I call it a negotiation, but it isn't much of one. Commercial payers like insurance carriers and the government tell healthcare practitioners what they're willing to pay for. This concerns most every service, from a blood draw to a heart transplant. Healthcare providers must work with that amount. This becomes a real problem when the cost of services increases as dramatically as it has over the last decade and a half, most acutely in the past three years. At its heart, the issue is that the expense side has increased far more rapidly than the revenue component, throwing the whole system into chaos."

A dot-connector by nature, Hallett points out other trends contributing to systemic stress due to so much economic mismatch. Practitioners opening surgery centers constitute one such stressor.[4] As he explains, "Certain services are leaving hospitals, such as the opening of orthopedic surgery centers. These are essentially doctors doing outpatient surgeries in their own facilities, choosing the patients they wish to see. Typically, these serve better-paying patients covered by commercial payers. So not only must the hospital they used to perform surgeries face higher costs, because of greater fixed costs with facilities, structure, staffing, et cetera, including traveling nurses from other areas, but they are also losing profitable procedures and services to these separate practices and specialized care centers."

According to Hallett, two primary causes are largely responsible for the economic woes of hospitals and healthcare systems across the nation. The first factor is high inflation.[5] "Over the past 30 years, technology like TVs and computers fell dramatically in price even as these wares grew more operationally powerful," says Hallett. "Healthcare has gone in the *opposite* direction. The industry is so overpriced to the point it's now the most expensive increase—percentage-wise—over this period."

The second factor is the cost of caring for America's aging population.[6] Hallett explains, "The average macro cost in treating an American up to about age 54 is roughly the same as in other first-world countries. But past that age, costs go through the roof. Certainly, we are practicing cutting-edge medicine the rest of the world later benefits from, but *because* we're first, it's the priciest. Meanwhile, as baby boomers remain the largest generational demographic, the exorbitant expenses for our older citizens become ever more acute."

In Hallett's view, such economic imbalance is the leading driver of our healthcare crisis. Medical malpractice lawsuits and insurance remain popular discussion points, but they are only minor contributing factors to the unfolding catastrophe.[7] Hallett explains, "When I was still at the University of Nebraska Medical Center, we started turning away 'regular' births and shrinking our obstetrics department to handle only high-risk births. That wasn't an issue of malpractice costs. It was because the reimbursement for regular births could not cover our costs. We literally had to tell OB-GYNs: 'Please don't come here. Go to the community hospital west of Omaha.' Birthing economics drove that decision. It wasn't malpractice insurance or lawsuits." Hallett also cites the increasing number of rural hospitals that have closed birthing centers for the same reason. "The problem for certain services and procedures is only growing."

Economic challenges facing hospitals and healthcare providers have led to an explosion in mergers and acquisitions to fix balance sheets. The University of Pennsylvania notes this trend led to a drop of 2,000 hospitals across the country, from 8,000 in 1998 to 6,000 in 2021, something Hallett believes will only continue.[8] Unfortunately, many such mergers do not achieve desired efficiencies. "In my experience, healthcare mergers, especially in the nonprofit sector, tend to result in few people losing their jobs. A merger's utility should come from the fact you now only need *one* hospital records staff—not two. Yet too often this fails to materialize in practice."

So far, we've established how economics largely drives our healthcare crisis. Now for the more critical question: How does this affect patients?

Is Patient Care on Life Support?

Recall Michael's struggle obtaining the specialist care his son needed for his allergies. In Hallett's view, patients in rural areas must now expect to drive long distances to receive such medical attention, the exact situation the Ashleys faced.[9]

Hallett puts this in perspective, "Our healthcare crisis is one of *efficacy*. And one of the major causes is lack of access. Americans in rural areas must now venture dramatic distances for specialist care or go without. No easy feat, it's especially difficult when the patient is ill or has a condition that makes travel uncomfortable. But what if I told you what we're seeing is no longer consigned to *rural regions*? Suddenly, urban Americans are up against the same shortfall. If you live on one side of a major city and the only specialist is on the other side, you're suddenly dealing with similar suboptimal care and all the attendant hassles rural Americans have put up with for years."

It isn't just patients feeling the pinch, either. Fewer capable American students are choosing to enter the medical field.[10] This phenomenon is partly due to high stress levels, not to mention the tendency to suffer burnout among physicians and other healthcare practitioners.[11] To many a young person contemplating a future career, the thought of practicing medicine seems like a losing proposition.

As Hallett explains, "The cost of education has emerged as a significant barrier to potential doctors and nurses, often costing us our best and brightest. The price of medical school has shot up so much that the only way some people can hope to complete their education is by taking on huge debt.

"And as we know, this burden will follow them throughout their lives. No wonder we have such a shortage of frontline general practitioners. Think about a student considering their future. When contemplating the massive debt they may accrue, they'll likely say to themselves: 'I better become an oncologist.' That's because many don't think they'll ever get ahead—even on a general practitioner's salary. Now add to that the stress and burnout factor, and we're all but pushing people with potential to be great doctors into other fields."

But Telemedicine *Can* Help

Despite so much bad news, Hallett believes things can still turn around.

He sees telemedicine's ability to not only deliver optimal outcomes to more patients but also help the healthcare industry overcome its existential crisis. In particular, he views telehealth as an exceptional tool, enabling Americans to enjoy the care of specialists as Michael's family did, leading to vastly improved health outcomes for patients across the board.[12]

"Telemedicine is all about speed and access," says Hallett. "Speed because it eliminates so many steps for both doctors and patients to come together. Access because it removes barriers for a patient to see a specialist. Much of our telemedicine conversation concerns primary care situations, but we can unlock its true power when we talk about specialists. There are tremendous advances to be made in so-called *doctor-to-doctor telemedicine*."

For starters, telemedicine can help patients stay local instead of having to travel to see a specialist. "Right now, the University of Nebraska Medical Center is doing groundbreaking work in transplants for small children," says Hallett. "Miracle surgeries, they transplant vital organs, such as the small bowel. It's easy to imagine a child living five hours away or more from their surgeon and specialists. If this same child happens to run a fever after successfully getting a transplant, their local physician or their hospital staff may think to put them in a helicopter or ambulance back to the transplant center for specialized treatment. *Is that even needed?* The local physician and/or midlevel provider, with all good intentions, practices such defensive medicine because of their own lack of knowledge and experience with such a complicated case. There aren't many options without direct communication with specialists at the academic medical center. *Now is this the best idea for the child?* Probably not . . . a specialist with years of experience and wisdom will likely say to the child's parents: 'You can treat this with over-the-counter painkillers,' then send them home. Okay. What if a general practitioner in rural Nebraska consulted with a specialist via telemedicine, removing needless transport hassles? Now you're getting somewhere!"

Hallett also recognizes the unique benefits of telemedicine outside of sheer convenience and the ability to extend specialist availability. "Many patients are intimidated by even entering a doctor's office. They may feel shamed by conditions like a sexually transmitted disease or addiction. Telemedicine removes fear of public exposure because patients remain safe and secure in their home, or in their car, or anywhere with an internet connection."

Our healthcare policy expert also notes telemedicine is an important component to tackling the crisis in mental health and addiction worsened by the COVID-19 lockdowns.[13] According to Hallett, "If we take mental health treatment and addiction care and place them in the same bucket, it becomes quite clear there are not enough providers and not enough available services. Anything that quickly expands providers and services to those needing help is a big positive. I so often hear people lamenting our many 'other' challenges in healthcare, but I will take these challenges over lack of access every single time."

Yet even when access *is* available, social stigma—for instance, the kind around opioid addiction—leads sufferers who desire help to avoid treatment. John Kelly, PhD, professor of addiction medicine at Harvard University and the founder and director of the Recovery Research Institute at Massachusetts General Hospital, explains: "People who feel more stigmatized are less likely to seek treatment, even if they have the same level of addiction severity. They're also more likely to drop out of treatment if they feel stigmatized and ashamed."[14] The cruel irony of addiction treatment is that patients feel stigmatized even when seeking treatment, such as the fear of being recognized by friends, coworkers, or family upon entering an addiction treatment facility.

Telemedicine, in Hallett's opinion, greatly lessens such negative feelings. "By definition, remote-based treatment for addiction is private. Confidential. The patient needn't worry about hiding the fact they are seeking support. It's also typically less intimidating than visiting a doctor's office. Besides, younger healthy Americans may have never required regular doctor visits, so the thought of attending a clinic weekly or monthly can be scary. By contrast, they may use video chat programs on their phone daily."

Telemedicine also offers significant benefits to practitioners. According to Hallett, "Whenever I've spoken to caregivers about telemedicine, they very much consider it to be a burnout antidote. For one thing, it reduces the need to commute. Without all the clutter and logistics of an office torn away, such as the ripple effect of a patient showing up late, they can spend even more time with patients. The best way for physicians to avoid experiencing fatigue is to ensure they can be with each patient long enough to make a difference. One helpful bonus to telehealth is that the doctor can also now achieve a desirable work-life balance they never could have dreamed of before."

Despite so many positives, Hallett knows challenges remain to widespread telemedicine adoption. Differing laws and licensing requirements persist, along with a protracted battle for telemedicine services to be fairly reimbursed by commercial payers and the government.[15] Despite these setbacks, he remains upbeat about telehealth's potential to solve our healthcare crisis.

"Telemedicine's downsides represent but a tiny percentage of the upside this approach provides to patients and caregivers alike," says Hallett. "Already, remote care offers so many Americans newfound access and immediacy. It's creating positive results in ways we don't completely understand. It's also the easiest solution to a large problem. It doesn't solve everything, but it puts a dent in our crisis, and that's unbelievably important."

Now that we can better appreciate so many positives in theory, let's drill down further. It's time to consider practical applications of using telehealth at the scale Hallett and others would like to see in the coming years.

CONVENIENCE MEANS BETTER CARE FOR ALL

The conclusion to Michael's story at the start of this chapter had a strong expediency element. Rather than spending precious time, energy, and the cost of visiting multiple doctors in two states to get relief for his son, the Ashleys found they could manage care from their home. All thanks to telemedicine. But as discussed, telehealth's convenience isn't limited to the patient.

To explain how the same concept applies to physicians, consider the case of a surgeon we'll call Dr. Majhi. Dr. Majhi specializes in repairing hernias. Restoring patients to full health, enabling them to enjoy physical activities like sports and exercise as they did before their injury, energizes our young doctor. What *doesn't* energize him? All the other hassles accompanying his job.

Many days Dr. Majhi makes the drive from Marin County (where he resides) to San Francisco (where he works), not to scrub in to the operating room and repair hernias, but rather to perform the many follow-ups after surgery. Putting in one and a half hours or more in the car—each way—just to spend five minutes looking at perfect sutures on his patients that don't fall into any risk groups is a waste of time. At least in Dr. Majhi's mind. He accepts this "grunt work" is part of the profession but wonders why it must be so painful.

Then one day Dr. Majhi learns of a fellow surgeon who uses telemedicine to make his day less galling. Specifically, his colleague relies on it to manage his routine follow-ups. (Certain patients like the elderly are rightfully earmarked for special attention and are always seen in person.) Intrigued by the idea, Dr. Majhi launches a pilot program to gauge how this approach might benefit his practice.

It's immediately a smashing success. Those young, healthy athletes Dr. Majhi typically operates on aren't required to come to the office. Neither is their progressive doctor. Instead, he performs follow-ups using patients' own smartphones to view the incision area. Batching time between routine appointments and surgery boosts productivity. No more needless suffering. Now, Dr. Majhi can see additional patients—and spend greater quality time with each one. Suddenly, his drive to work isn't so bad. If he must drive in, it's for surgery or to provide a higher level of care for his at-risk patients.

Several considerations emerge from Dr. Majhi's tale. First, his overhead is bound to go down. A smaller staff can handle all the appointments, allowing him to downsize his office to save on rent or mortgage. He also saves hours fighting traffic and locating a parking spot daily. From an organizational perspective, missed appointments fall to unprecedented levels.

But what about Dr. Majhi's patients? They love the new arrangement. Not long ago, some would blow off their surgical follow-ups. Now they only must take their smartphones out of their pockets. Overwhelmingly positive about telemedicine, many leave five-star reviews since Dr. Majhi switched to remote. Plus, a few patients he treated at a local nonprofit hospital made donations after their great experiences under this new model. Within months, Dr. Majhi proved telemedicine can be a win for the physician, patients, and even hospitals.

SAVING ERS FOR REAL EMERGENCIES

A study by researchers at the University of Maryland School of Medicine proves a rule of thumb in healthcare: when Americans need medical help, many don't shy away from visiting the emergency department (ER). In fact, they head for the ER about half the time they believe they need care. African Americans are the likeliest to go to the ER, with 54 percent considering it their preferred provider. That figure climbs to an astonishing 59 percent in urban areas.[16]

Dr. David Marcozzi, author of the University of Maryland study and an associate professor of emergency medicine, believes this is a matter of quality healthcare availability. "This research underscores the fact that emergency departments are critical to our nation's healthcare delivery system. Patients seek care in emergency departments for many reasons. The data might suggest that emergency care provides the type of care that individuals actually want or need, 24 hours a day," he writes.[17]

Randall Hallett believes this is another area where telemedicine can shine. "If those seeking care from the emergency department that aren't in a true crisis can turn to telemedicine, several things happen at once. First, it gets less expensive for all parties. Second, they're likely to get immediate attention instead of a long wait. Third, they're not taking their family members into an environment where they might get sicker. There's nowhere worse to go to get ill than the ER."

The net result? Better care for all, but African Americans in particular, because of their increased likelihood of going to the ER for frontline medical care. Overall costs fall. And wait times for the seriously ill and severely affected plummet. Meanwhile, physicians and ER staff are less stressed. They can focus on the most desperate cases of injury and illness detrimental to true ER patients.

SPECIALIST ACCESS WHEN THE CLOCK IS TICKING

Sometimes a delay in accessing specialist care isn't just a matter of feeling miserable for a longer period, like Michael faced with his son's allergies. Sometimes, a treatment delay can create a ripple effect, devastating a child's development for years to come. One such case concerns autism therapy.

The number of children diagnosed with this disorder has soared in recent years.[18] According to the CDC, the autism rate in children has reached 1 in 54, including an astounding 1 in 34 boys.[19] A mom we'll call Alice believed her son Jack to be exhibiting indicative signs. Eventually, he was diagnosed with autism spectrum disorder (ASD) at age three. She wanted to find the best option to help her son successfully manage ASD. Instead, she learned the demand for autism therapy far outstrips current supply.

Knowing how early intervention is key to helping Jack achieve his full potential, Alice devoted her time to finding the best medical option. Her research led her to applied behavioral analysis (ABA), a widely respected and recognized therapy. After devouring several books, research papers, and even YouTube videos on ABA, she was enthusiastic to get Jack started.

Here she ran into a problem much like Michael's experience with allergists. There was only one ABA provider in Alice's hometown. This person informed her she would have a four-month wait to even have her son undergo an assessment. Frustrated by the long wait and worried about how such a delay would affect her son's chances to lead a healthy life, Alice sought alternatives.

Alice considered long drives to a provider in another state. This proved impractical based on time and expenses. She also contemplated private care she'd pay for out of pocket. It was just as unaffordable as traveling long distances. Like so many Americans, she hadn't considered telemedicine for Jack because she knew little of its existence. But then the idea came to her as an offhand suggestion from a family member who said: "My cardiologist offers telemedicine appointments. Maybe autism specialists do too."

Alice latched onto telemedicine options, fast locating a children's specialist with proper credentials and relevant experience. Highly rated for both in-person and telemedicine treatment, the provider could offer the exact same service level to Jack as if she lived in their city instead of five hours away. Instead of waiting four months for a basic assessment, Jack began ABA therapy just two weeks after Alice located the telemedicine provider.

Soon, Alice could already see marked improvements in Jack's behavior and activity level. He responded well to ABA, quickly learning new skills to help him achieve academic success. When Alice's ABA provider told her Jack's prognosis was strong for flourishing in a mainstream school setting, Alice knew she'd made the right decision by getting her son immediate help instead of waiting for a local provider.

WHEN THE MAYO CLINIC ISN'T NEARBY

The Mayo Clinic built its reputation on a groundbreaking multidisciplinary healthcare approach.[20] More providers now emulate the Mayo Clinic model, but this method can collapse in the face of specialized medicine. As discussed by Hallett, most young doctors want to be a specialist these days because of stark economic incentives. Our economic system favors the highly specialized, like pediatric oncologists, over general oncology. Yet extreme specialization creates tremendous friction for patients: for one, the need to see a specific specialist to get needed treatment.

Yet as we've seen, not everyone lives in Manhattan or the suburbs of Chicago, where there appears to be an unlimited supply of specialists.

So how can patients living outside these areas ever hope to tap into the knowledge and experience of leading providers? For those who cannot afford a private jet and/or an extended hotel stay to seek the perfect specialist, the overwhelming answer is telemedicine.

In later chapters we explore remote care's potential, both for today and for tomorrow. But first we must examine one key by-product of our healthcare crisis—burnout for doctors and their many harried patients.

CHAPTER 6

The Great Resignation Comes for Doctors and Nurses

Candace, a 36-year-old medical doctor (MD), sat at an empty table in the back of a hospital cafeteria. She ate cold soup from home without even tasting it. In her heart, she felt she *should* be happy about her career and her life. A prestigious healthcare provider, she worked her dream job as a plastic surgeon. She had two beautiful kids with her husband, also a physician. Instead, she dreaded returning to work after this short break. Dr. Candace didn't have to guess *why*. Still, she worried it was a clear case of burnout, something toxic that had wrecked careers of colleagues in recent years.

Prior to this, Candace had her heart set on plastic surgery, ever since medical school. She worked hard throughout her education, standing out as a skilled surgeon dedicated to patients. While some future physicians in her classes scoffed at plastic surgery as "doing nose jobs for rich teens and breast augmentation for their moms," Candace knew her field's importance. It was her way to give patients a new lease on life. Every time she repaired a cleft palate, reconstructed facial bones after a horrific accident, or rebuilt deformities, she took pride in her contributions, giving others the chance to live a life they didn't imagine possible.

Clearly, Candace sounds like an engaged physician. *What went wrong?*

Before considering the factors leading to Dr. Candace's burnout, we must examine what this potential career killer entails. The Mayo Clinic defines burnout as "a special type of work-related stress—a state of physical or emotional exhaustion that also involves a sense of reduced accomplishment and loss of personal identity."[1] By 2020, the symptoms accompanying burnout read like a laundry list of Candace's daily emotions. Woefully cynical, she'd even grown overly critical of coworkers. Many avoided her for this reason (especially in the mornings). She also had to drag herself to work and often had trouble getting started. Constantly drained, she chugged ever more coffee to combat fatigue. Her rest cycles weren't spared, either. She had trouble drifting off and staying asleep. Random unexplained headaches also plagued her.

In short, she was miserable. The only time Candace felt like herself was when she was fully scrubbed up in the operating room. The bright lights, her team of talented specialists and nurses working beside her like a well-oiled machine, and most importantly, the patient relying on her to restore them to health could snap her out of her emotional doldrums.

Although she felt great in the OR, burnout had tortured Candace for two years by now. The workplace stress that wore her down will be commonplace to most physicians. Strain from juggling patient appointments and paperwork, occasional arguments with insurance companies who knew nothing about their customers (and cared for them even less), plus the need to forever do right for her patients—despite a troubled healthcare system—took their toll. But the biggest contributor to Candace's burnout? Her work-life *imbalance*.

For years Dr. Candace sacrificed time at home to make it in plastic surgery. She put in long hours, many spent far away from her true love, the operating table. Her husband is also a self-admitted workaholic.

When their daughter was born in 2015, both weren't around as much as they would have liked. Even now, she feels intense guilt over hiring an au pair to raise her little girl because of her hectic schedule. She missed so many milestones in her daughter's life. She despaired at how that would only worsen when her child went to school. *How do you make it to sports games and concerts when you're busy debriefing after an operation—or presenting a paper to a panel of peers in another state?*

Yet all these problems were but a prelude to what Candace experienced during COVID-19. If she thought her life and career were chaotic before the pandemic, late 2020 proved her utterly wrong. Working longer hours than ever, she subjected her family and friends to a higher risk of contracting coronavirus brought home from the hospital. The discomfort of taking daily COVID tests became a nightmare ritual. To make matters worse, she had to take a pay cut because of the number of surgeries she would normally perform being ruled "elective" out of her control.

It seemed that the operating room, her one oasis of happiness, was now a smaller part of her career than ever. But the factor that drove her to the brink of crisis had nothing to do with the hospital. In early 2021, Dr. Candace learned she was pregnant again. This time, she was having twins. Once she got over the shock, all she could think of was how uncertain her future just became.

She asked her husband, "Can my career survive this?"

He didn't have a clear answer.

The couple knew she would have to take off *at least* three months for maternity leave, hurting her professional prospects. Likewise, having three children to care for instead of one—and two of those being very young—complicated the family's childcare situation. Candace knew she wanted to be more involved in the twins' early lives than she had with their older sibling—while also getting more engaged with her firstborn. Truly, she felt like she was facing a quandary: *Can I be there for my kids—and my patients? Must I choose*?

For a whole week after learning she was pregnant, Candace treated her patients with utter competence, as usual. Still, questions about her future swirled around her brain. *Must I pick family over patients?* She kept debating. In time, Candace told friends, both inside and outside the hospital, about her pregnancy and career concerns. Sympathetic to her plight, many advised her to stick it out. But one HR executive had a different idea and sent Candace an email with the intriguing subject line, “Maybe there’s a third option?” Candace’s pal had sent a link to the employment site Indeed.

Candace clicked to see what this person had in mind. The link went to an ad from QuickMD seeking telehealth providers. Her initial reaction was to dismiss the idea outright. *I’m a plastic surgeon!* she thought. *Zoom can’t help me treat patients.* But she trusted her friend’s instincts, so she put more thought into it. Her thinking evolved to *I’m a burned-out surgeon not operating on patients—and not making an income worth being away from home.*

Realizing telemedicine could be a viable future, she researched the possibility in earnest. She talked to her network about their knowledge of telemedicine in general and QuickMD specifically. She heard positive things and was shocked to learn a doctor she’d assisted with multiple patients had already made the leap. She spoke to the current QuickMD doctor over lunch. She was struck by how comfortable he seemed. If that physician’s demeanor was anything to go by, telemedicine could be her lifeline. Yes, she would have to switch away from plastic surgery, but still, the pros could outweigh the cons.

Finally, after much soul searching and discussions with her husband, Candace applied to become a care provider with QuickMD. Her life changed. For the better. Candace’s average day with QuickMD now unfolds much differently. She no longer starts well before 8:00 a.m. and ends long after 5:00 p.m. She also no longer has a difficult commute to and from the hospital. Better yet, she drastically cut back on her au pair's hours. That's because she now spends so much more time with her three cherished children.

Most importantly, she's in control of her schedule. And her life.

Dr. Candace works the hours she wants to work. She builds a schedule to neatly fit around the twins' nap time, feedings, and that hectic 30 minutes when her husband scarfs down breakfast before heading out to his job. But the luxury of working remotely extends beyond controlling hours. It's a small thing, but she can dress more comfortably and wear less makeup, which she always felt was more for the benefit of her colleagues than her patients—especially when the latter was unconscious on an operating table.

Like the colleague who answered all her questions about telemedicine and QuickMD, the impact on Candace's stress level was both dramatic *and* immediate. She found she could get the same thrill of success through telemedicine as she did in the operating room, especially when she became qualified to treat opioid addiction. Every time she connected with a patient suffering from such compulsion, she felt the same surge of satisfaction helping them achieve a better life as she did working as a surgeon.

Candace continues to enjoy success in telemedicine ever since joining QuickMD. As COVID-19 restrictions have lessened, she's even found opportunities to return to the operating room, typically assisting doctors in procedures she is quite experienced in, rather than taking the lead (plus all the accompanying grunt work). Two years after eating cold soup she couldn't even taste in an empty cafeteria, Candace now enjoys lunch daily with all three of her children. Moreover, she feels revitalized as both a mom and a physician, and she owes it all to the telehealth revolution.

THE PROGNOSIS ON BURNOUT SHOULD SCARE US ALL

Having read Dr. Candace's fictionalized story, we encourage you to poll others who don't work in healthcare about physician burnout. That's what we did, randomly sampling people in our lives, asking them, "What percentage of physicians do you think suffer from this?" Although our informal polling efforts were not the most rigorous, we think you'll find similar answers yourself. On the low end, one respondent stated he thought only 10 percent of doctors face this problem.

Overall, the consensus figure for physician burnout came in at about 33 percent, with the high estimate being 45 percent. That figure isn't too far off the mark for the *pre-pandemic* era—which seems like the distant past.[2] But for all the damage caused by COVID-19, what many aren't talking about is the epidemic of physician burnout associated with it. The *actual* levels of doctor burnout should be as concerning to Americans as the macro challenges to the healthcare system described in the last chapter.

The startling truth of our crisis came to light when the *Mayo Clinic Proceedings* published the work of doctors who surveyed fellow physicians from around the nation to assess their burnout, work-life integration (WLI), depression, and professional fulfillment. The figure that should get the metaphorical crash cart rolling is the burnout number: 63 percent, or almost *two out of every three* physicians surveyed.[3] They all reported at least one burnout symptom. You may have read Candace's tale believing she was an anomaly. According to this research, she represents *the average doctor in America*.

To this point, Dr. Tait Shanafelt, oncologist at Stanford University and leader of the cadre that performed the research, explained, "It's just so stark how dramatically the scores have increased over the last 12 months."[4] Bryan Sexton, director of Duke University's Center for Healthcare Safety and Quality, told the *New York Times*: "This is the biggest increase of emotional exhaustion that I've ever seen, anywhere in the literature."[5]

Clearly, burnout is a far more serious problem than most realize—with the exception, perhaps, of the stressed physicians themselves, and those healthcare professionals who work with them. Burnout has been a hot topic for years, including a National Academy of Medicine report issued in 2019.[6] Yet the survey by Shanafelt and colleagues found that burnout is particularly difficult for physicians in the COVID-19 era because of the tendency for it to be combined with other challenges.

The second important part of the survey focused on work-life integration. This term can be used interchangeably with work-life balance, but the two have distinct meanings.[7] Work-life balance concerns establishing designated "work hours" and separate personal time where work is not to be performed. Doctors have long known work will often intrude into personal moments, so the survey instead focused on *integration*, ways in which we artfully blend together work and personal tasks, such as Dr. Candace making lunch for her kids while catching a Zoom presentation. Even with the survey's emphasis on integration over balance, the numbers for American doctors are on life support.

Only 30.2 percent of doctors surveyed reported feeling satisfied with their work-life integration (WLI). That's less than one-third who feel good about their WLI, extra worrisome when you know doctors go into the profession thinking their career will gobble up a staggering amount of time. Simply put, there isn't a physician or nurse who came up through the legacy healthcare system who expected their job to be a comfortable nine-to-five occupation. So even with the *expectation* they will be working a huge number of hours, more than two-thirds are now throwing up their hands in frustration. In Dr. Candace's case, this breakdown in WLI was most noticeable in her relationship with her daughter and concerns about her twins.

One natural question to ask is: Are doctors feeling bad about work because *everyone* else seems to be feeling bad about work? As it turns out, the COVID-19 pandemic was a challenging time for all working Americans, not just physicians. Yet an argument could be made that doctors are more depressed because working Americans are more depressed. But depression levels among physicians were only a *part* of the survey published in the *Mayo Clinic Proceedings*. The results show that general depression is not the culprit. Depression increased by a modest 6.1 percent among physicians.[8] (Once upon a time, a 6 percent rise in depression among doctors might have raised eyebrows, yet when placed in the context of catastrophic numbers for work-life integration and burnout, a small depression increase is little more than a blip on the radar!)

Even so, the relatively small bump is important. It tells us the problems doctors face are due to their jobs, not their mental makeup. As the authors explain, "Notably, the differences in mean scores for depression at the end of 2020 and end of 2021 were modest, suggesting that the increase in physician distress in this interval was primarily due to increased work-related distress."[9] It also shouldn't be a surprise that as burnout and the disintegration of WLI have occurred, job satisfaction has flatlined.

According to the survey, the percentage of doctors who demonstrated high professional fulfillment scores dropped from 40 percent in 2020 to just 22.4 percent in 2021. That's a collapse of nearly half in a single year. Only 57 percent of doctors in the survey said they would be a physician again if they could go back in time.[10] Does this sound like a prescription for a healthier America? To us, it's an unmitigated disaster. To make matters worse, it represents a veritable healthcare crisis hitting some physicians and patients worse than others.

Of course, doctors have never been a monolithic group, moving in lockstep. The problem of burnout and work-life integration becomes especially thornier once we recognize how doctors working in different specialties experience different stresses and strains on their mental well-being, just as male and female physicians undergo disparate workplace challenges. (You'll recall that a contributor to Candace's own burnout was the fact many surgeries she would have performed during the pandemic were canceled, causing her income to plummet as her general workload skyrocketed.) Although not necessarily for the same reason, the survey found burnout is particularly bad for emergency medicine, family care, and general pediatrics. This matches the observation of coauthor Dr. Omer, himself an emergency medicine physician.

Just as burnout affects practitioners differently based on specialty, it also affects doctors based on gender. The survey shows women physicians are more likely to suffer the strain than men. The authors suggest one explanation, writing, "These data suggest that the long-documented increased risk for burnout and work-life conflict in women physicians has been exacerbated by the COVID-19 pandemic, a finding consistent with other reports."[11]

The "long-documented risk" they refer to has been studied for almost a decade, with research completed in 2014, 2020, and 2021 all generally finding female physicians suffer from lower work-life integration satisfaction—putting them at greater risk for burnout—than men.[12] In Candace's case, she felt guilt for not fulfilling a traditional maternal role for her daughter, and also expected serious troubles keeping up with her career once she had twins. For many other female doctors, it may not be a matter of childcare, but simply the constant onslaught of hours and on-call nights that finally wear them down.

The study by Shanafelt and colleagues also delivered a sobering conclusion in the calm language we might expect from an academic work. It is nevertheless frightening enough to keep healthcare leaders awake at night. Consider their carefully chosen words as they describe the scope of the problem they've exposed:

> The COVID-19 pandemic has exacerbated preexisting problems in the health care delivery system and taken a dramatic toll on the US physician workforce. A striking increase in occupational burnout and decrease in satisfaction with WLI occurred in US physicians between 2020 and 2021. Differences in mean depression scores were modest, suggesting that the increase in physician distress was overwhelmingly due to work-related distress. Given the association of physician burnout with quality of care, turnover, and reductions in work effort, these findings suggest that ongoing efforts to mitigate physician burnout are critically important for the US health care system. Timely, system-level interventions implemented by government, payers, regulatory bodies, and health care organizations are warranted.[13]

Dr. Jack Resneck Jr., president of the American Medical Association (AMA), echoes the authors' sentiment. He says that the "sober findings" from the post-COVID research should be used to take "urgent action" to combat physician burnout, including "supporting physicians, removing obstacles and burdens that interfere with patient care, and prioritizing physician well-being."[14] We agree with Dr. Resneck, which is why telemedicine and its ability to remove or mitigate many of the worst burnout causes must be a prominent component of any plan. Otherwise, how can we expect doctors like Candace to do their best work with patients daily?

DOCTORS AT THE END OF THEIR ROPE

Most physicians suffering from burnout eventually conclude they have two options. Option one: Stay in the medical field, hoping things will improve. This can take the shape of moving to a new location, like across the state line. Yet even this approach typically requires they grit their teeth and bear it. Option two, especially for women of childbearing age who want a family, like Candace, is to step away for months, years, or maybe forever. This choice has major societal negatives. For starters, we are left with one less doctor to treat our aging population.

As for Candace, telemedicine presented a third option. Instead of continuing on as she had, or outright quitting, she began practicing in a new way, one better fitting her desired work-life balance. Knowing more about why doctors suffer burnout and the work-life integration failing so many of our caregivers, the ease of transitioning to telemedicine makes sense for those in Candace's position. Working remotely, physicians like Candace no longer must spend long days toiling in a hospital or a busy office. They are also spared a mind-numbing commute to work and back. Better yet, Candace was able to reduce her au pair's hours, spending more time with her kids, including attending her daughter's first dance recital. Finally, Candace could integrate her work with her family life. For example, she can choose to not see patients at 3:00 p.m., as this is when her twin babies wake from their nap.

When Candace joined QuickMD's ranks, she met other physicians who were also bouncing back from burnout. They joked about celebrating the end of their professional nightmare with a party and cake, as if it were a birthday. Along the way, she encountered other capable physicians who weren't burnt out but still felt forced out of the legacy healthcare system because of the increased schedule crunch and expected grunt work. For instance, one of Candace's new coworkers is missing a hand.

It's much easier for her to work at home using a special keyboard and mouse setup she is most comfortable with. Another colleague suffers from an eye problem preventing him from looking at his computer screen for more than an hour at a time. That could have been a death blow in the legacy healthcare system, but at QuickMD it is a minor scheduling matter.

Ultimately, telemedicine offers a viable career path for physicians suffering from burnout and for others who are increasingly finding the legacy healthcare system incompatible with their work-life balance or other needs. The danger to the healthcare system is that many physicians in the same predicament as Candace still see their choice as binary—suck it up or leave altogether. To better understand the threat of doctors resigning at scale—a potential catastrophe for our collective health by any metric—we needn't look further than what's occurred in the economy across multiple sectors—a.k.a. the Great Resignation.

"TAKE THIS JOB AND SHOVE IT"

Starting in 2021 and extending through the present, a jarring phenomenon has emerged. It's puzzled economists, business leaders, and even organizational psychologists. Millions of Americans are voluntarily vacating jobs. According to *Harvard Business Review*, 57 million Americans quit between January 2021 and February 2022.[15] Names like "the Big Quit" and "the Great Reshuffle" have also been thrown around to label this marvel, but the moniker that stuck was "the Great Resignation," coined by Anthony Klotz, professor of management at University College London's School of Management, in an interview with Bloomberg.[16]

Speaking to the *Harvard Gazette*, Harvard professor of economics and labor economist Lawrence Katz explained, "I think we've really met a once-in-a-generation 'take this job and shove it' moment." Katz expanded on his startling statement with his view of the Great Resignation: people's financial situation is stronger than it was at the end of the Great Recession, and they are more likely to request remote work and question "low-wage, high-turnover situations."[17]

Helpful insights to be sure, yet perhaps the best source of info about the Great Resignation comes from the individual who correctly forecasted and named it—professor Anthony Klotz. Klotz shared his view with *Business Insider* in a 2021 interview. Klotz predicted that serious career burnout, especially in the service sector, would lead to mass resignations. He discussed how people's identity can be tied to their career and position and how interrupting that—through work-from-home, a layoff, or quitting after burnout—can help people experience life more fully.[18]

In another comment particularly applicable to those doctors who have been on the frontlines of the COVID-19 response, Klotz says that "when human beings come into contact with death and illness in their lives, it causes them to take a step back and ask existential questions. Like, what gives me purpose and happiness in life, and does that match up with how I'm spending my right now?" In some cases, those reflections lead to life pivots.[19]

Yet Klotz also sees a silver lining to the Great Resignation. He believes it is a unique chance for employers to transform their relationship with employees to create a new normal, one that works better for both parties. He told *Business Insider* he hoped the COVID-19 pandemic would create permanent focus on employee well-being.[20]

We agree with this assessment.

But it is even more critical for doctors to have a healthy and sustainable career, free from burnout and impossible work-life imbalances. We also believe the costs to our country presented by the Great Resignation possibly spreading to more doctors (and don't forget nurses) are so serious they must be avoided at all costs. Thankfully, telemedicine offers an ideal way for doctors suffering burnout and other vocational stresses, to such a degree that they are considering a career change, to keep their talents where they belong—helping patients achieve healthier lives.

More importantly, we don't believe telemedicine is merely some replacement for a career in a hospital or a brick-and-mortar office. Instead, remote-based care offers a variety of unique benefits that when combined make for a strong resource for *both* doctors and patients whose needs are not being met by the legacy healthcare system.

BETTER PATIENT RESULTS

Speaking of patients, it should be clear by now how telemedicine acts as a viable replacement for the typical visit to a doctor's office. It provides untold benefits, like not waiting to see a physician in a room full of sick people, avoiding trouble finding a specialist, and saving time *and* money. But for other patients, and also from the business/economic viewpoint of providers, telemedicine has outsized potential to improve lives, making the United States a healthier country.

Telemedicine's diversity, flexibility, and innovative applications create situations whereby patients benefit. Often, this takes the form of unique physician relationships that might be hard or impossible to achieve in legacy healthcare. For example, QuickMD's TeleMAT treatment for opioid addiction includes several physicians who are themselves recovering addicts. Their ability to provide care while expressing firsthand knowledge of what they went through has been profoundly impactful.

Second, telemedicine's national pool of doctors provides patients with a vast array of personalized care. And because patients are now no longer limited to their local area, they can find a doctor who looks like them, someone with the background to take them seriously, or even someone with training in alternative forms of medicine, such as traditional Chinese medicine (TCM). To this point, at QuickMD, one of our physicians is trained in both Western and Ayurvedic medicine, a traditional healing practice from India.[21] Can a patient expect this diversity from their local doctor?

Third, telemedicine's ability to move fast opens up possibilities for treatment with cutting-edge medical sciences. For example, the *Harvard Health Blog* has documented emerging therapies using ketamine for the treatment of major depression, traumatic brain injury (TBI), and other mental health disorders.[22] In the legacy brick-and-mortar healthcare system, a patient that doesn't live in one of the few cities that has already opened a clinic featuring ketamine treatment may have to wait years to discover if this innovative protocol might become available. If telemedicine becomes an option for ketamine treatment? They will have their answer in days or weeks instead.

BETTER PROVIDER RESULTS

Many telemedicine advantages are also available to physicians, some of which mirror those received by patients. Staffing a telemedicine company is a whole new ball game for some of the same reasons listed previously. Employers can now tap into a national candidate pool. Also, no longer are hiring decisions so reliant on doctor availability by region. The question becomes: What doctor is the best fit in our *country*? Likewise, increased capital flows are pouring into tech and staffing, as there is little to no need for brick-and-mortar facilities, with all the expenses they can incur.

Another telemedicine benefit for providers? Suddenly, they have *happy* doctors on their hands. Free from debilitating burnout and the daily grind so many caregivers see as standing between them and their patients, remote physicians feel more engaged with their work and purpose. Reflecting on her first month in this new arrangement, Candace found she spent more time talking to patients, helping them achieve positive health outcomes—all without worrying about needless busywork piling up on her desk. To be sure, happy doctors make fantastic employees, as is the case with every type of job.

Flexibility in scheduling offers yet another boon to providers. When telemedicine doctors want to work long shifts, it's often because they are engaged and interested in their work, not because they are desperately trying to cover the overhead of their office. Likewise, given the flexibility to choose hours, some physicians will happily take night or weekend shifts, as those fit their schedule preferences. Better yet, when doctors don't feel crushed by the hassles of day shifts—and then night and weekend hours added on top—their performance and engagement improve at the same time providers reap the benefits of improved patient service and efficiency.

At the end of the day, telemedicine isn't a total cure-all. As stated, there are still many areas of medicine we don't predict telemedicine will handle anytime soon, such as trauma care or childbirth. There are also multiple hoops to jump through, like licensing requirements that can vary by state. And of course, there are regional pharmacy issues.

Yet, despite these hurdles, telemedicine undoubtedly helps doctors, patients, and providers in groundbreaking ways. Every month, more and more physicians are rescuing their careers from burnout and stepping back from the ledge of the Great Resignation. They are also rediscovering their love for medicine through telehealth. And for every doctor that joins the telemedicine movement, thousands of patients are finding increased levels of care and treatment they believed to be unreachable, especially after languishing in the legacy healthcare system.

In the next chapter, we explain how QuickMD got started in the first place. We also demonstrate how the six pillars of telemedicine guide everything we do.

CHAPTER 7

Our Story

Although legal documents give his name as "William J. Smith," everyone in the rural West Virginia county where this takes place knows the man at the center of our tale as "Little Bill." Little Bill stands at six foot five. He also clocks in at over 275 pounds, yet his nickname isn't some ironic nod to his size—like Robin Hood's right-hand man, Little John. No, Bill got his nickname after his father, also named William—known as "Big Bill."

Unfortunately, Big Bill died when Bill was just 14.

A blue-collar guy, Big Bill long held a "work hard, play hard" mentality. The "play hard" part had to do with heavy drinking, going back to his teen years. By the time Little Bill was a kid, his dad had become a full-blown alcoholic. Big Bill even turned to stimulants far stronger than coffee to go to work in the morning. Little Bill knew his dad had a drinking issue. But he had no clue his family was about to go through a nightmare because of it.

By the time Little Bill reached 14, he had four younger siblings, two who were very young. Even now, he can recall the Friday night his father died. That's because he tried to keep his dad from going out that evening. Little Bill's siblings were already asleep at the time. Their dad was supposed to take all the kids fishing the next morning.

Unfortunately, Big Bill had just gotten paid. He was ready to raise hell with his friends. Like many payday parties, this one was all but guaranteed to devolve into an all-nighter, leaving him passed out when he should have been helping Little Bill and his siblings bait hooks with nightcrawlers. Knowing all this from past experience, Little Bill charged out of the house as soon as Dad fired up his Chevy truck. "You can't go out tonight. You promised to take us fishing tomorrow."

Big Bill just grinned with eyes glassy from drinking for hours before ever entering his first bar. "Listen here, son. We're just going out for a quick drink or two to unwind. I'll be back in no time." His pal Steve cackled in the passenger seat at the obvious lie.

Little Bill had gotten this kind of brush-off before. He didn't buy it. "You're drunk *already*."

Big Bill started to say something nasty but thought better of it. He hadn't been drinking long enough to let his mean side come out. "Well, I've had a few, but let me let you in on a little secret . . ."

Little Bill waited.

"The secret to life is to control the booze—instead of letting it control you. Now run along and we'll all have a good time tomorrow. You wait and see."

With that, Big Bill tore off into the night.

Little Bill and his siblings didn't have fun the next day. Bill's father ran his truck off a bridge that night, killing himself and Steve. The accident changed the course of Little Bill's life, in the same way Little Bill's life would take a dramatic turn 20 years later.

But first, after Big Bill passed, the family plunged into poverty.

Mom tried to support her five kids, but it was a struggle to keep them fed and clothed, even with government help. Back when Little Bill was finishing high school, any dreams of going to West Virginia

State for football flew out the window. As the oldest sibling he now had to support his brothers and sisters.

Little Bill landed a job in a factory after graduation. He worked his way up the ranks. Before long, he was a certified forklift driver, a position of importance in any factory or warehouse. He also stayed clean, not using any drugs or alcohol throughout his high school and adult years. Unlike friends and coworkers, who typically picked up the drinking patterns of their father or drug habits plaguing the state, his dad's demise galvanized Little Bill to never touch the stuff. Daily, he got up for work with a clear head and thought, *I'm not like Big Bill and never will be.*

By his early thirties Little Bill was married with two children and thriving. Uncommon skills on the forklift plus a knack for leading others sent him up the career ladder. It also provided his family a comfortable life that was a far cry from the poverty he and his siblings had endured. He was doing everything right.

Then fate intervened. He suffered a serious work accident. One day while Little Bill was moving equipment, a junior operator ignored safety regulations. Taking a blind turn at a reckless speed, he slammed into Little Bill's forklift. When the shock wore off a second later, Little Bill thought he was okay. But then intense pain like he had never felt before shot up his right leg.

Something was very wrong.

The accident had caused Little Bill's foot to jam down on the brake pedal with tremendous force. Either steel from the assembly or the bones in his foot had to give way. As you'd expect, Little Bill's foot lost that confrontation. He suffered a Lisfranc dislocation,[1] along with multiple broken metatarsal bones.

En route to the hospital in an ambulance, Little Bill worried the accident would be ruled his fault, blemishing his spotless safety record.

He needn't have fretted. There was no question the other driver was to blame.

The junior operator was found to be high on opioids while working, a fact that would become cruelly ironic given what would happen to Little Bill.

Little Bill underwent emergency surgery to fix the dislocation. This involved inserting metal pins to hold everything in place. "You'll have to wait a month for the follow-up," said the doctor. "Then we can fix the broken bones in your foot when the swelling and inflammation have gone down. This should help you in the meantime." He gave Little Bill a prescription for OxyContin, advising his patient to get plenty of rest and to remember to elevate his foot.

Little Bill didn't like this at all. He recognized the name of the drug as an opioid he'd heard about on the news. "Doc, I don't use drugs. Is this really the best medicine for me?" The doctor waved away his concerns. "This is a new painkiller, and the manufacturer says it's rarely addictive. As soon as that surgical numbing agent wears off, you'll want those pills. But trust me. You'll be fine."

Little Bill did as told.

The pills did dull the pain and make him feel good. But by the time he was ready for follow-up surgery, Little Bill's OxyContin was now a lifeline. He'd take one in the morning; go to work, where he was assigned desk duty; and then count the hours until he could take the next dose as his foot became more painful.

He did not know it, but Little Bill's habit was forming.

Soon after, he underwent a four-hour surgery to fuse his broken bones. This left him with screws and a metal plate embedded in his right foot, and a fresh OxyContin prescription. This time, he didn't argue with the doctor. Little Bill was grateful to have a fresh prescription (with refills!)

from a professional who seemed more than happy to throw opioids at even the slightest discomfort. And Bill couldn't afford to miss more work.

Recovering from his second surgery, Little Bill's opioid habit intensified. OxyContin became an indispensable part of his routine. Yet he didn't view the pills as a drug to get high. He thought of them as a necessary part of his healing, enabling him to get back to work full time on the forklift.

But Little Bill also noticed he required more pills for the same effects.

Whenever he tried cutting back, he struggled with the pain. The plate in his foot burned hot inside his flesh. And sometimes he felt other old injuries, like throbbing in his shoulder from his football days. Even weirder, his mind seemed to be playing tricks on him, as the pain would mysteriously shift to his other foot. This phantom hurting scared him, but not as bad as the time he tried to cut OxyContin out of his life.

Even after Little Bill could walk normally again, he still clung to the OxyContin. Though part of him worried he was putting himself and coworkers at risk by driving a forklift on drugs, he counted on his skills to keep safe. At the same time, he was growing increasingly worried by his addiction. *I can't end up like Dad*, he thought.

That's when he vowed to stop using cold turkey.

Only things didn't go so well for Little Bill. He soon felt sick all over, sweating, with agonizing foot pain. He believed this to be at least partially phantom pain, but that didn't make it easier. His muscles cramped and twitched, blocking out all thoughts. And of course, he couldn't sleep a wink that night. He just lay awake counting the hours until shift time, desperately wondering if he would ever be healthy again.

After that horrid night, he ran to OxyContin like a drowning man to a life preserver. *This is just to get through my shift*, he told himself. Providing for his family was more important than fixing what he considered to be a minor inconvenience. But opioids weren't that—they were swallowing Little Bill whole, putting him at grave risk for leaving his own kids in the same nightmare Big Bill's alcoholism had left Bill and his siblings.

Months went by. Little Bill was now back in the office for a checkup. The same doctor said he was pleased with the condition of Little Bill's foot. "A complete recovery," he pronounced.

But Little Bill wasn't exactly walking on air.

After the examination, Little Bill ventured the question he'd rehearsed on the drive over. "Um, Doc, that's great and all, but do you think you could write me a fresh Oxy prescription?"

The doctor put down his chart. "But you don't need medication anymore. You've made a full recovery."

"Yeah, but—"

"You shouldn't need anything more than a Tylenol for a tough workday."

Little Bill felt uncharacteristic anger. "Listen here, Doc. I took those pills 'cause *you* said they're safe. Now I agree they're safe. And I need them."

"Little Bill, I don't think that—"

"I told you. Write me a prescription now!"

From there, things got out of hand. The argument reached fever pitch. Gone was Little Bill's composure. Instead of just screaming, he stuck his finger in his doctor's face, making frightening threats.

By the time the medical office manager came to see what was going on, the doctor had his phone out, dialing the police.

Little Bill left in a panic.

At least he still had 10 OxyContin left. *That was something*. But not enough. He needed a prescription to re-up his supply. That worried him. But not as much as the thought of trying to kick his addiction. Shuddering, he recalled how sick he had felt the one time he'd gone off drugs.

So he started making calls. Before long, he found a friend of a friend willing to sell him a few pills from his own stash. This black-market foray launched what Little Bill later referred to as his low point. For months, he went from person to person, buying up opioids. First acquaintances. Later strangers with legitimate prescriptions, all to feed his cravings. Beyond the shame he felt lying to his wife ("No, honey; I quit the pills ages ago"), one stark downside to this approach was money. It fast became costly to keep himself supplied.

Little Bill soon knew he needed a cheaper way to satisfy cravings. (Though he never thought of it that way—he still considered what he was doing as "treating pain" or "avoiding problems.") No matter what he called it, this is when he turned to street drugs.

By now, Little Bill knew many others using, or more correctly *abusing* opioids. He'd traded pills with them throughout his county. He also knew many of these addicts who similarly needed cheaper highs had turned to heroin. In fact, about 80 percent of heroin users first misuse opioids in pill form.[2] Even so, needles scared Little Bill. His pursuit of a cheaper high led him to fentanyl, something very cheap, especially when pressed into pill form.

For all his risk-taking up to now, Little Bill was still no fool. He knew fentanyl was dangerous. He'd heard about it on the news for years. Still, he thought he could handle it. He was dead wrong.

The second day he took his new drug of choice, he overdosed. He felt different right after taking the pills. Little Bill's breathing slowed as his vision dimmed. Sitting in the driver's seat of his car parked in his driveway, he sensed himself sinking into a deep hole. He lost consciousness. Luckily, his neighbor, a paramedic by trade, happened to notice. He saved him with naloxone, a medication to rapidly reverse opioid overdose.[3]

"Little Bill," said his neighbor, shaking his head afterward. "I keep naloxone in my car because I run into folks OD'ing wherever I go.

But I never expected to have to use it in my own neighborhood. You need help."

"I'm fine," said Bill.

Even he didn't believe his own words. All Little Bill could think about is what his dad told him the night he drove off that bridge: "The secret to life is to control the booze instead of letting it control you." Little Bill had lost all illusions by now. He knew that just as Big Bill couldn't control alcohol, he couldn't control opioids. He needed help, and he didn't know how to get it.

Little Bill and his wife first considered an addiction clinic administering methadone. But going there required a two-hour drive on a daily basis. And everyone would know his business if he showed his face there. Also, methadone didn't appeal to Little Bill. He worried it wouldn't be safe for workdays. His research brought him to another option, medication for addiction treatment, or MAT.[4]

The more he read, the more he grew interested.

As mentioned in chapter 4, MAT uses a combination of buprenorphine, itself an opioid, and naloxone, the latter which saved his life by blocking the drug's effects. When combined, most commonly under the brand name Suboxone, these medications effectively treat opioid addiction. They reduce cravings while smoothing out withdrawal effects. If a patient happens to take an opioid, Suboxone limits the effect, thanks to the naloxone in it. This all sounded fantastic to Little Bill, but there was no provider anywhere in his area.

He worried he was out of luck until his wife stumbled across something. Googling MAT providers, she found an option neither knew existed—TeleMAT, an addiction treatment powered by telemedicine. Specifically, she found a discussion of people endorsing it as a "lifesaving" and "life-changing" option. Both Little Bill and his wife knew of telemedicine from using the service for their child's ear infection, so Bill planned to call after work.

Desperate for help, he hoped he'd found the answer to his prayers.

Hours later and from the privacy of his home, Bill brought up QuickMD's app to start his appointment. After a brief wait, he connected with QuickMD's coauthor and cofounder, Dr. Omer. Feeling anonymous using his online connection, Little Bill described how he had hit rock bottom. Dr. Omer recognized familiar patterns from patients he'd served. Looking him up in West Virginia's prescription drug monitoring program, Dr. Omer also learned Little Bill's doctor had cut him off.

Not long after Bill had turned to street drugs, he now had a prescription for Suboxone waiting at his pharmacy. As a new patient, Little Bill received one week's worth of medication. After that, he could get a stable supply after a follow-up visit. Although Little Bill's story is fictional, it mirrors those of countless patients, many of whom credit Dr. Omer, QuickMD, and TeleMAT for helping them break their addiction.

Key takeaways from Little Bill's experience with QuickMD can be summarized this way: He could start his recovery in a healthy way, supported by a doctor. He could quickly see a prescribing physician when hospitals and clinics were shut down during the COVID-19 pandemic. His appointment fit his schedule and lifestyle. Finally, his addiction treatment was private, devoid of stigma.

HOW LITTLE BILL'S STORY FITS TELEMEDICINE'S SIX PILLARS

Little Bill's triumph over drug abuse using QuickMD and TeleMAT demonstrates core strengths of the telemedicine platform our team built. It's also an excellent illustration of the six pillars we laid out earlier.

Let's take a moment to review these, examining how they apply to Bill, not to mention so many more others suffering from opioid addiction.

Pillar 1: Enables Greater Access

As a reminder, this pillar is met if the increased pool of providers offers greater patient access to care. This pillar represents the clearest need for telemedicine when confronting addiction. Little Bill wasn't as concerned with finding his ideal provider as he was with finding *any* MAT resource. The only addiction clinic in his area required a lengthy drive and relied solely on methadone treatment. Surprisingly, MAT access is often limited, even in suburban and urban areas—not just in rural sections like this sparsely populated West Virginia county.

Pillar 2: Promotes Stronger Patient Follow-Through

This pillar is fulfilled if the telehealth delivery model results in higher patient adherence rates. Again, Little Bill couldn't adhere to his doctor's recommendations if he couldn't find a doctor offering MAT treatment with Suboxone in the first place. As a secondary aspect of this pillar, a key component to Bill's recovery has been the privacy telemedicine affords. The social stigma of seeking addiction treatment contributes to a low adherence rate,[5] but there is no dishonor in telemedicine. No one is likely to know about it unless *you* tell them.

Pillar 3: Desired Care Exceeds Need

This pillar exists if telemedicine eliminates inefficiencies by providing immediate appointments. Imagine a scenario where Little Bill has access to a doctor who offers MAT, but the real barrier isn't the distance or travel time—it's the lengthy wait to get into the service. For mental health and substance abuse treatment, the wait can be excruciatingly long. The average wait time for a first psychiatric appointment can be several weeks to months, and for specialized services requiring specific expertise or skills, it can extend even longer. In Little Bill's case, even if a doctor was available for treatment, the agonizing wait for initial access or follow-up care could have severely hindered his recovery process. This highlights a critical inefficiency in the healthcare system that telemedicine aims to address, making timely care more attainable and reducing the excessive delays too many patients face.

Pillar 4: Removes Barriers

Pillar 4 applies if telemedicine speeds up medical treatment without incurring negative effects. For individuals battling opioid addiction, these obstacles are not only geographic but also psychological and societal. The first significant hurdle is the geographical scarcity of addiction specialists, particularly in regions most affected by the opioid crisis. This physical distance makes it challenging for many, like Little Bill, to find available treatment options, such as medication-assisted treatment (MAT). Beyond tangible distances, there are intangible yet profound barriers, such as the intense social stigma associated with seeking treatment for addiction. The mere act of walking into a clinic can feel like a public admission of one's struggles, deterring many from seeking needed help. Telemedicine offers a discreet and accessible alternative, effectively removing these visible and invisible barriers. It also provides a private, stigma-free channel for patients to reach out for help, thereby broadening access to essential healthcare services.

Pillar 5: Expedites Care

Pillar 5 is met if telemedicine speeds up medical treatment without incurring negative effects. Little Bill could see a QuickMD doctor within minutes of entering a virtual waiting room. He chose to have his appointment at the end of the day, but he could just as easily have engaged with the app during a lunch break. Now, contrast such convenience with having to coordinate an appointment at a traditional healthcare facility. The latter would likely involve taking a half or full day off work and then wasting time driving to the clinic, before sitting in a waiting room. On the other hand, when seeing a doctor is easy, care is helpfully expedited, and recovery can begin.

Pillar 6: Enables Wellness

This pillar is met if telemedicine empowers patients to optimize their health without negative consequences. Little Bill's TeleMAT treatment optimized both his health and the health of others. First and foremost, it hastened his entry into recovery. His addiction didn't worsen. It also didn't produce more misery for his loved ones. Instead, he could see a telemedicine doctor fast, getting better sooner than he believed possible. Of course, TeleMAT also benefited the health of the entire community, mainly because of what *didn't* occur.

Since Little Bill could get off dangerous opioids and on his road to recovery, he did not cause a workplace accident or some other disaster. He avoided dangers so often caused by drugs that would have likely affected others—like his dad's car wreck. He also didn't hinder first responders and an ER trying to save his life after overdosing again. Little Bill's recovery meant he wasn't adding stress to an already strained healthcare system, especially amid the COVID-19 pandemic.

Little Bill's story and those of thousands of Americans just like him are the reason why QuickMD's leadership and growing team of physicians so enthusiastically embrace telemedicine. It was also our own personal brushes with tragedy that led us to build a novel solution to our opioid crisis.

Fortunately, a loosening of telemedicine laws borne out of necessity during COVID-19 allowed our team to present patients like Little Bill with lifesaving TeleMAT. But part of the QuickMD story concerns how we were even in the position to act on these legislative changes in the first place. This is because our systems and services were *already* built out and working before the pandemic. In fact, the seeds of QuickMD were planted back in 2015.

A TRIO OF FRIENDS' SCRAPPY START-UP

Some fledgling companies have leadership teams assembled by venture capital investors and other outside influences. While QuickMD has worked hard to recruit optimal talent to flesh out our organization, our core leadership team comprises three friends with an unlikely story of meeting. Together, we found common ground in our drive to revolutionize healthcare, using tech to connect doctor and patient.

Before this venture, Chris Rovin and Jared Sheehan partnered in PwrdBy, a firm committed to social and environmental impact via innovation, data science, and software design.[6] They engaged in cutting-edge projects, such as producing an app for 150 children's hospital systems and creating a carbon emissions calculator for major multinational corporations. But their true passion involved applying our skills to helping others, and to addiction in particular.

This passion led us to enter a 2015 FDA innovation challenge on fighting opioid abuse and its severe health consequences. Our winning entry was a prototype to automatically deliver naloxone to those suffering an overdose. (Such a device could have saved Little Bill if his neighbor hadn't found him in his driveway.) The project seriously impressed the consulting physician assigned to our team: Dr. Talib Omer.

Our prototype held the potential to save lives, and a follow-up proposal was accepted by the National Institutes of Health to put it into production; unfortunately, no funding was available. We therefore decided to transfer the idea to Brave Co-Op, an organization engaged in preventing opioid overdoses.[7] No matter. Chris, Jared, and Dr. Omer hit it off. The foundation of our friendship involved our mutual interest in combating opioid addiction—an interest intensely personal for all three of us.

Each QuickMD cofounder has a connection to addiction and overdoses. Jared was shaken by the death of a baseball coach and high school classmates who passed after overdosing on illicitly purchased opioids. Chris had multiple friends overdose, with some living and some dying. And Dr. Omer worked in the ER where he saw an endless stream of broken lives and devastated families: from overdose cases rushed in via ambulance, to car wrecks caused by high drivers, to people in recovery sitting hours in the ER hoping to get a Suboxone refill to avoid becoming another grim statistic.

As an ER physician dealing with opioid fallout on a regular basis, Dr. Omer understood MAT and Suboxone were safe and effective for patients. He also knew many physicians perceived Suboxone to be similar to methadone, a strong opioid that must be carefully monitored and administered by a clinic. Many naysayers believed Suboxone could never be prescribed via telemedicine because of the mistaken belief that it was just like methadone.

Yet every day that Dr. Omer spent in the ER—seeing multiple people successfully apply MAT—convinced him that MAT via telemedicine, or TeleMAT, *could* be an effective solution. Yet regulations controlling telemedicine and MAT held him back. Even so, he envisioned what QuickMD could be.

BRINGING QUICKMD TO LIFE

Dr. Omer knew he had several options after medical school.

He could go the traditional physician route, contributing to society's betterment. Already, he was making a name for himself working as an assistant professor of emergency medicine for the University of Southern California in the West Coast's largest county emergency department. The other option? Challenge himself. He'd always felt an entrepreneurial spirit. He'd even launched his own nonprofit app, which now has over 5 million downloads, on top of managing his busy, stressful career in emergency medicine.

By mid-2019, Dr. Omer's constant musings on telemedicine's ability to help people who spent miserable hours waiting to be seen in the ER could no longer be shoved into the background. It was time for telemedicine to take a leap forward, and he knew just who could help him do it. He reached out to his friends Chris Rovin and Jared Sheehan.

Chris and Jared helped Dr. Omer establish the technological infrastructure that would become QuickMD. Chris built its first marketing website in August 2019. And Dr. Omer saw the company's first patient in October 2019. It was a man seeking a doctor's note for work following a lingering illness. Dr. Omer estimates he saved the man from hours of needless running around just to prove to his employer he was sick—time better spent resting in bed. The patient was thrilled with the help.

More importantly, QuickMD was born.

THE SHIFT TO ADDICTION CARE

QuickMD wasn't in the business of treating addiction for its first six months because government regulations wouldn't allow it. Instead, it served as an online urgent care, helping parents get help for their sick children, assisting workers with doctors' notes, and treating all sorts of maladies with social stigmas, such as sexually transmitted diseases. This all changed in March 2020, when telemedicine regulations loosened and Dr. Omer could at last bring his vision for TeleMAT to life.

During the early months of QuickMD, Dr. Omer juggled his ER shifts with running the business and seeing most patients himself. Back then, QuickMD didn't have an office. He therefore managed operations and saw patients from his dining room table—while leveraging a strong internet connection.

Things changed between March and October 2020. Dr. Omer now oversaw a team of seven doctors he knew previously and had invited to join QuickMD. Soon, he shifted to a purely management role as a curious thing happened: demand from patients *and* physicians eager to join the QuickMD revolution exploded.

HOW QUICKMD REACHED 200 DOCTORS

As our start-up picked up steam, we knew we needed more doctors. Surprisingly, one of the best referral sources came from current physicians. We offered a bonus for each new doctor we'd hire, but we almost didn't need to. QuickMD doctors felt a sense of purpose while enjoying a flexible work-life balance. As a result, they've become experts at spotting physicians in their circles who could benefit from the same arrangement.

Despite the speedy pace of so many excellent referrals, we also posted ads to attract new doctors, especially as we expanded into new states.

The following is the text of an early job description, one of the first things a physician exploring telemedicine would see as they sought out career opportunities:

> QuickMD is a rapidly growing telemedicine service that is looking for friendly doctors to join our team (IM, EM, Family med) for at least 16h per week. Apart from regular urgent care-type patients, we have lots of patients that need monthly refills of their buprenorphine/Suboxone to avoid opioid relapse. Therefore, an X-waiver (XDEA) is required. We are busy, and you will be able to see enough patients in your shift to make $100 per hour completely remotely, with flexible hours.
>
> Please note that since March, the DEA allows and encourages Suboxone to be prescribed via telemedicine and we are trying to do our part to increase access to MAT. These are very rewarding patients to take care of.
>
> We pay above industry standards (16–25% more than the largest telemedicine companies) at $35 per consultation, and the average consultation time is 8 minutes and rarely goes up or beyond the allotted 15 minutes (work notes, STD treatment, UTI treatment, and refills of buprenorphine are about 90% of the cases).
>
> Because of the current reciprocity, we are seeing patients in most of the country, but the majority are in California.
>
> Minimum Requirements:
>
> - Medical license in California or at least the temporary COVID-19 emergency license for California
> - Completed or almost completed residency in IM, EM, or family med

- Requirement to work at least 16 hours per week (mostly early afternoons starting at 12p and any time on weekends, as well as some M–F mornings)
- Be open to complete a ~4-hour online addiction provider training (paid by QuickMD) as lots of our patients are on buprenorphine and need regular refills (X-waiver)
- Excellent bedside (website) manners, friendly and knowledgeable around common urgent care complaints

Malpractice insurance provided. Last month our 18h/week docs saw on average 247 patients (=$8,645). 1099 provided at the end of the year.

While our volume can be high, and it can get quite busy during your shifts, we can disable the "on-demand" feature for your shift if you desire and only allow 1 patient per 15-minute time slot if you so prefer.

We are using a secure and easy-to-use custom telemedicine platform.

It isn't hard to notice this job description includes information about compensation. Many doctors are skeptical they can earn a good living in telemedicine. Their view of the service is limited. They perceive it to encompass the occasional urgent care product for healthy families. Doctors (and we don't blame them) prefer the security of a $200,000 salary instead of no salary—and a payment-per-patient-visit model.

Accordingly, many physicians expect to start telemedicine slowly, thinking they must build a book of patients as they would in a legacy model. But the typical physician who joins QuickMD is shocked by patient demand. Many see five to six patients an hour and 30 to 50 a day, earning $35 per visit. Some see 80 patients a day because they find it rewarding and don't have the scheduling concerns of a young mom, for example.

When doctors learn they can make an excellent living without the work-life strain, commute, and a thousand other trifling problems of working in a doctor's office, clinic, or hospital, their financial concerns disappear. Upon realizing they can make life easier for multiple patients an hour, helping them overcome addiction—or even save them hours seeking care for a common concern like shingles—they're sold on a new career with QuickMD. Many of our physicians feel the shift to telemedicine is the best thing they've ever done careerwise. One example is Dr. Robert Stern, who we first hired part time and is now our chief medical officer, leaving behind his roles as the medical director of the Addiction Medicine Clinic at Johns Hopkins and as a medical officer with the State Department in the U.S. Foreign Service.

The story of QuickMD's astonishing growth centers on the confluence of several factors. These include:

- The government relaxing telemedicine restrictions during a global crisis
- A common cultural familiarity with internet services like Zoom
- Recent breakthroughs to create effective, customized software to run a medical business

But most of all? QuickMD's surprisingly quick success is due to three committed friends who saw the role telemedicine could play in revolutionizing the American healthcare system. We are especially honored to bring hope to patients like Little Bill who suffered so long from opioid addiction.

Now that you know how we got here and how our story fits into the wider healthcare picture, let's visualize the future of health—all from the convenience of your smartwatch.

Read on to find out.

CHAPTER 8

Wearables, Telehealth, and the Path to Rapid Response

If we were to ask you to name one actress who made a huge mark on pop culture, who springs to mind? We coauthors tossed this question around and came up with diverse answers. One author mentioned Sigourney Weaver. She demonstrates unbelievable versatility, moving from the heroic Ripley in *Alien* (1979) to a comedic turn as Dana Barrett in *Ghostbusters* (1984) and then combining both in *Galaxy Quest* (1999). Yet another proposed Zendaya. She stole the show as the fierce warrior princess Chani in *Dune* (2021). But for sheer impact on the zeitgeist, not to mention an indelible tie-in to the near-term future of telemedicine, there's a sleeper who must be considered.

Her name? Edith Fore. We always get the same reaction: "Who?"

Not knowing Edith's name is understandable. She wasn't a trained actress. She also was never featured in a Hollywood film. What did she do? She appeared in a commercial. *USA Today* called it the ad "that left the most indelible marks on our collective memory."[1] Edith Fore is responsible for a phrase that spread through American culture long before the internet made memes a part of daily life.

Edith is the woman who once said: "I've fallen, and I can't get up!"

Her ad that would become a media juggernaut was commissioned by LifeCall, a company with a device we would today call a "wearable." The equipment included a pendant a senior who might become incapacitated could wear. This allowed them to communicate to a helpline via a wireless connection to a base station installed in their home. Think of it like a cordless landline but through a bauble worn around one's neck.

At its heart, the idea was to use modern tech to avoid an all-too-common tragedy: seniors found dead in their home after a fall rendered them incapable of seeking help. When they set out to make their TV spot, LifeCall had the idea to use a real customer's experience with the service. Little did they know they were about to create something so unique it captivated a nation. It also provided endless fodder for late night hosts' jokes, as well as spoof commercials.

Edith Fore, a retired school nurse, was in fact a LifeCall customer.[2] The incident portrayed in the ad is a dramatization of an actual situation where she used the LifeCall radio transmitter to summon help. In fact, it's fair to say the commercial is a scaled-back version of the truth to make it TV suitable. *Deseret News* describes her 1989 accident as a fall and head injury that left blood dripping into her eyes.

The fact the LifeCall pendant offers a single button for emergencies must have been a crucial feature for her summoning assistance. As Edith told the *Phoenix New Times*, "They needed someone who had actually used the system." Yet, when the producers laid out the situation for the commercial, including a fall, she initially declined the offer. As she stated, "I told them I wasn't interested because I'd taken enough falls in my lifetime."[3]

LifeCall said they would provide her a stunt double. This person would fall, instead of requiring Edith—in her 70s at the time of filming—to collapse before the camera. Another interesting fact about the commercial? The iconic line "I've fallen, and I can't get up!" comes from Edith herself. She explained in an interview that writers created the scenario based on her accident before adding, "But that line is mine."[4] What came next was a cultural phenomenon.

As the *Phoenix New Times* explained in 1990:

> Since the commercial first aired last summer, the pathetic cry has turned up as a message on tee shirts and telephone-answering machines and has provided material for standup comedians and at least two novelty records. Earlier this month, the irritating wail even inspired a star-studded party deemed "downtown New York's event of the season" by *USA Today*. The voice behind this much-mimed mantra? One 74-year-old Edith Fore, easily the unlikeliest candidate for fame since the late Clara Peller brayed "Where's the beef?" in a series of Wendy's commercials.[5]

Edith's famous line would even make an appearance in a parody ditty by "Weird Al" Yankovic.[6] Meanwhile, sitcoms like *The Golden Girls, Family Matters, Roseanne*, and *The Fresh Prince of Bel-Air* also referenced it. Gary Larson even immortalized it in a *Far Side* cartoon. (Back in the pre-internet era, this was the equivalent of being the top trend on Facebook, Twitter, Reddit, and YouTube—all at once—and for a shocking bout of time.)

Long before most families had even a basic internet connection through America Online, seemingly *everyone* knew the LifeCall ad. Now, normally any company would be over the moon to enter the cultural milieu in such spectacular fashion. For one thing, it multiplied the ad campaign's impact through free exposure to consumers.

The problem for LifeCall is that seniors, its target market, weren't in on the joke. One company spokesperson told the *Phoenix New*

Times, "It's our generation and the college kids who are picking up on this commercial. If you ask someone who's a senior, they're not aware of the craze because it's the Arsenio Halls, the Johnny Carsons and the . . . Howard Sterns who are using the line."[7] Edith didn't get rich off the craze either—she received only a one-time payment for the wildly successful ad.

Still, the LifeCall ad created a pop culture craze persisting to this day. The Internet Meme Database has an entry on the phrase to explain it to millennials and Generation Zers born long after the commercial hit airwaves.[8] While it is an interesting story in its own right, we feature the tale as an intro to tech solutions with potential to revolutionize telemedicine. That technology is today called wearables—and LifeCall offered a crude early version previewing so many latter-day devices promising to revolutionize healthcare.

WHAT A DIFFERENCE 30 YEARS MAKES

NPJ Digital Medicine, published by *Nature*, provides us with this definition for such novel innovations. "Wearable technology, also known as 'wearable devices' or simply 'wearables,' generally refers to any miniaturized electronic device that can be easily donned on and off the body or incorporated into clothing or other body-worn accessories."[9] In the modern era, the wearables concept comes with the assumption they include powerful computing power or at least the ability to communicate with a smartphone or other device.

Of course, the LifeCall pendant wasn't a smart device. Neither were Bluetooth and Wi-Fi part of the daily lexicon. Even so, the device served a purpose. It empowered seniors facing true medical emergencies. Yet by definition, LifeCall and similar devices were *reactive*. An accident or health crisis would occur, and then the senior would have to use the pendant to call for help. There's a major assumption baked into this process—that the individual is conscious *and* able to activate their wearable device. In many cases, especially those involving head wounds, seniors could not take that assumption for granted.

Now, just over 30 years later, we have entered the era of *proactive* wearables. Today's tech affords us the capability to constantly track patients and monitor their well-being in real time. Put it this way: Imagine if Edith's wearable device knew she had taken a serious fall *before* she could even think about summoning help. How much more helpful would that be?

For a more extreme example, imagine a wearable capable of predicting a heart attack before it happens based on tracking blood chemistry and other biometrics. Such early intervention might well stand between life and death in many cases. In fact, wearables are advancing so rapidly they now offer the same level of monitoring previously only possible in a hospital setting, a subject we explore in greater depth later in this chapter.

THE (ALMOST) WEARABLE PRACTICALLY EVERYONE POSSESSES

Strictly speaking, a smartphone isn't a wearable. Still, they're about as close as a device can come to being one, given how many of us keep our phones within reaching distance at all times. According to a recent poll by YouGov, 31 percent of Americans can't go more than a few hours without their phones. Another 17 percent wouldn't want to go a full day without their device. That's almost 50 percent of the population who might suffer a meltdown without access to their smartphone for just 24 hours. Naturally, 46 percent of those surveyed agree with the following statement, "Not having my phone with me makes me feel anxious."[10] Given their vaunted status as a "close-to-wearable" device, smartphones currently present interesting opportunities to explore the potential for wearables to proactively monitor our health.

Of course, smartphones *already* play a central role in telemedicine. Most QuickMD patients connect to their physician using an app on their Apple iOS or Google Android smartphone. No matter the device, each has a basic health monitor out of the box. The Samsung Health app for Android smartphones can also track steps taken by monitoring the phone's movement, although it may not be as accurate as a dedicated fitness tracker.[11]

But it's a recent software innovation that provides an interesting comparison to the old reactive wearables' approach. With the launch of Apple's iPhone 14, the company added a new feature titled Crash Detection. It's designed to sense car accidents and summon help in case of an emergency. MacRumors, a website dedicated to in-depth reporting on Apple and its products, describes how when the Apple Watch or iPhone detects a crash, an alert displays for 10 seconds.

> If you're still responsive, you can swipe the screen to call emergency services immediately or dismiss the alert if you don't need to contact them. If after 10 seconds you haven't interacted with your Apple device, a 10-second countdown will start. When it ends, emergency services are contacted.[12]

To reiterate, Apple's Crash Detection monitors data for signs of an accident and then contacts first responders if the user doesn't respond to prompts confirming they are okay. Unlike LifeCall and similar systems that could once upon a time only summon help if the user could activate it, the new Apple feature will call in the cavalry *unless it's waved off.*

For a young Indianapolis man, Crash Detection meant the difference between life and death. Nolan Abell was wearing a recently purchased

Apple Watch when he suffered a car accident in October 2022. The event, just months after the app launch, serves as a demonstration of wearable proactive alert devices. According to ABC News, Abell ran into a pole after losing control of his vehicle while driving too fast. Stunned, he struggled to stay conscious and was disoriented by the collision.

One thing in the vehicle wasn't disoriented—his Apple device. Within seconds of impact, Abell felt his watch buzzing, asking if he was okay. When he didn't respond after 20 seconds, it summoned emergency services. Abell later told ABC, "If it weren't for this watch, who knows how long it would have been for help to get to me. Someone would have found me eventually, but this had EMS to me in five minutes."[13]

Such technology offers obvious applications for close monitoring of seniors and other at-risk populations. If our phones and watches can detect a car accident, it's a mere matter of turning them on to detect someone falling down the stairs, a common household accident involving the elderly. Even so, active monitoring like Crash Detection *does* require a balancing act from device makers and service providers. There is always a risk of false alarms—especially when so many adventurous activities can mimic a car crash.

As an example, the *Wall Street Journal* noted in 2022, around the time of Abell's accident, how roller coaster rides often set off Apple's Crash Detection.[14] The high-G source of excitement can trick devices into thinking a user has suffered a serious accident when they were only at risk for throwing up a greasy amusement park lunch. As seasons have progressed, the Crash Detection has also mistaken falls on ski slopes as serious incidents worthy of emergency responses.[15]

There was a fivefold increase in false 911 calls from the Bonnaroo Music Festival in Tennessee in the summer of 2023, due to iPhones summoning help after mistaking dancing for a car crash.[16] Authorities sent messages to attendees asking them to disable the feature after a flood of calls caused chaos for first responders. Even so, many calls still had to be checked out by police officers. (Unsurprisingly, when 911 dispatchers called back dancing revelers unaware their devices had summoned emergency support, they couldn't hear a phone ringing over the blaring music.)

Despite these hiccups in Apple's tech, it's clear smartphones have a tremendous opportunity to work hand in hand with telemedicine. But they are just the start. An amazing array of innovation is occurring daily in the wearables space, with nearly every device offering a direct application to improving remote based care.

Beyond wearables, the same concept of passive monitoring found in Apple's Crash Detection is making a difference in the war against overdose deaths. Brave Technology Co-Op, which the QuickMD cofounders are investors in, produces overdose detection sensors for public bathrooms and other overdose hotspots to detect absence of movement, or depressed breathing, raising the alarm before a potential overdose can turn into a preventable fatal tragedy.

MORE THAN JUST FITNESS TRACKING

Fitbit, acquired by Google in 2021, is the most prominent brand in the crowded market for wearable fitness trackers.[17] Those interested in improving their health and activity levels enjoy the many features Fitbit provides, like heart rate assessing, step counting, even sleep monitoring. Like all good wearables, the Fitbit also efficiently communicates with a smartphone app to provide consumers with useful data in a clear, easy-to-read format.

But Fitbit has expanded from tracking fitness to something more dramatic. In 2017, *Today* reported on how 73-year-old Patricia Lauder credits her Fitbit with saving her life.[18] Patricia wore a Fitbit to track her steps, like many doing their best to maintain a physically active lifestyle. But the device contributed to her health in an utterly different way. After suffering from a sinus infection, Patricia found herself short of breath. A doctor's visit failed to provide answers, so she planned to wait it out.

Luckily, she kept checking her Fitbit stats, because the "wait it out" approach may have proved fatal. What Patricia found by examining her app was a disturbing trend in her resting heart rate. It had started at 68 beats per minute but was steadily climbing by 5 beats per minute daily. In a few short days, her resting heart rate was an astonishing 140 beats per minute, way beyond the normal range for a senior citizen.

By the time she called an ambulance she was turning blue from oxygen lack. Doctors quickly diagnosed her with a pulmonary embolism, or blood clots in her lungs. *Today* quotes Dr. JuYong Lee, who treated Patricia, as explaining, "If she had not looked at her heart rate maybe she would have neglected her symptoms and not come to the hospital. She may have died if she hadn't checked her Fitbit."[19]

Patricia's tale is an example of how wearable tech can save lives. Still, it relied on her checking her device's app to gauge her health data. Imagine the tragedy if she wore her Fitbit and it recorded her health information, but she didn't log in while not feeling well, so she never sought attention. This possibility must be something the engineers behind the device considered too, because the company is taking the next step into proactive health monitoring with updated features.

Wareable, the leading news site covering such tech, reported in June 2022 that Fitbit had rolled out a proactive monitoring feature.[20] (Many Fitbit devices are now capable of providing continuous passive monitoring to detect atrial fibrillation, commonly referred to as AF or Afib.) The condition centers on an irregular heart rate that can cause serious health problems.

As explained by a paper published in the *Journal of Geriatric Cardiology*:

> Atrial fibrillation (AF) is the most common arrhythmia diagnosed in clinical practice. The consequences of AF have been clearly established in multiple large observational cohort studies and include increased stroke and systemic embolism rates if no oral anticoagulation is prescribed, with increased morbidity and mortality. With the worldwide aging of the population characterized by a large influx of "baby boomers" with or without risk factors for developing AF, an epidemic is forecasted within the next 10 to 20 years. Although not all studies support this evidence, it is clear that AF is on the rise and a significant amount of health resources are invested in detecting and managing AF.[21]

Continuous passive monitoring for AF is a tremendous leap from the monitoring that saved Patricia's life. It also has the ability to warn of a problem *before* reaching a crisis. That's exactly what happened to New Orleans DJ George Ingmire. Ingmire, 54, bought a Fitbit for the same reason as most people—to increase his activity levels, enhancing his health.

But one day the app gave him a warning about AF. He compared this alert to a car's "check engine light" in an interview with a local NBC station.[22] When he went to a cardiologist to later confirm the Fitbit's message, Ingmire discovered he did have a serious case of AF, and surgery was needed. Without his Fitbit, the problem might not have been discovered until he suffered a stroke. Instead, he has a new lease on life.

Now, imagine how this tech could be applied to telemedicine. Heart rate data and active monitoring could go to your remote physician through a secure internet connection. This will give your doctor real-time info about your condition. Or maybe the AF detector will alert your caregiver at the same time it tells you, the wearer of the fitness tracker. Certainly, receiving an alert about your heart would be better managed with the help of a doctor's advice. Likewise, in Patricia's case, an active data connection with a telemedicine service might have saved her an ambulance ride and a scary brush with death. It's easy to picture her doctor contacting her with concerns over a rising heart rate long before it ever reached the critical stage.

Most importantly, the potential impact of Fitbit and similar heart rate trackers when combined with telemedicine is enormous. Moreover, it isn't something to be speculated about in some far-flung future—the technology is here *today*, and the use case couldn't be clearer. Continuous health monitoring needn't be limited to a few minutes in a frantic doctor's office or in an uncomfortable testing location. Instead, it can proactively offer the level of data needed to identify serious health conditions, often before they reach crisis levels.

Of course, there are still many unanswered questions about this tech. One concerns patient privacy. With constant streams of data flowing between device manufacturers and healthcare providers, how might privacy laws like HIPAA be properly followed? Beyond that, how might providers deal with data overload? Also, is it the provider's responsibility to provide monitoring around the clock? (It's easy to imagine a scenario where a device detects a potential stroke, but no one is on duty to react.)

These are important conversations to have as the technology evolves, but as you'll see in the following sections, what we've described until now is also far from the only effective health outcome wearables can offer from the telemedicine perspective.

MOVE OVER, MOOD RINGS

Wearables are evolving beyond the wristband. One popular device demonstrating the changing format is the Oura Ring.[23] True to its name, it is in fact a ring worn on the finger. Unlike the Fitbit and other wearables, the Oura Ring focuses on what our bodies can tell us while asleep. This is useful because in this state, we have little to no idea if we are suffering from sleep apnea and/or other common disorders with life-threatening consequences. On the other hand, sleep is of critical importance to maintaining good health.

Along these lines, Harvard Medicine explains the recuperative theory, describing why sleep is so vital:

> Another explanation for why we sleep is based on the long-held belief that sleep in some way serves to "restore" what is lost in the body while we are awake. Sleep provides an opportunity for the body to repair and rejuvenate itself. In recent years, these ideas have gained support from empirical evidence collected in human and animal studies. The most striking of these is that animals deprived entirely of sleep lose all immune function and die in just a matter of weeks. This is further supported by findings that many of the major restorative functions in the body like muscle growth, tissue repair, protein synthesis, and growth hormone release occur mostly, or in some cases only, during sleep.[24]

So how does the Oura Ring tackle the sleep issue? By tracking your body's physiological activity while off in a dream world. In a review of the device in *Shape* magazine, Oura CEO Harpreet Singh Rai explains that sleep is a good time to measure physiological things because we're not moving. He notes that the device's accuracy for resting heart rate during sleep is about 99 percent to that of an EKG.[25]

The device reports three scores that are easy to understand and to act on. It rates the wearer's physical activity during the day, their sleep quality, and their readiness for the next day. Beyond these surface metrics, the Oura Ring tracks other helpful variables, such as sleep latency, or the time it takes a wearer to fall asleep after their head hits the pillow. The device also measures important aspects of heart performance, such as heart rate variability (HRV).

Shape notes that the Oura Ring tracks resting heart rate (RHR) and HRV (how much time passes between each beat). "In general, a higher HRV is usually a sign that your heart is adaptable and your autonomic nervous system (which is responsible for the fight-or-flight response) is functioning well. And the lower your RHR, the more efficiently your heart is working." This capability is similar to that of another device, the WHOOP, which tracks various biometrics, including resting heart rate and beats per minute, overnight.[26]

Like the Fitbit, imagine the power of this data when paired with telemedicine. A patient can connect to a physician from the comfort of their home and have sleep data available for sharing instantly. In practical terms, this means no need to engage in a sleep study in some uncomfortable lab, no wasted time for patient and physician alike in trying to get test results, just immediate actionable data and fast, efficient answers to medical troubles.

As stated, the Oura Ring has potential to improve health outcomes when paired with telemedicine. But perhaps the greatest leap forward is available through Apple in the form of blood glucose tracking.

SAVING DIABETICS FROM A KILLER MILKSHAKE

Bloomberg reported in early 2023 that Apple has made big strides in developing tech to measure blood glucose levels without the need for diabetics to ever prick a finger.[27] The innovation will likely be introduced as a wearable in the form of the Apple Watch. This will measure blood glucose continuously through the skin. So far, Apple has developed this project in secret since even before the death of Steve Jobs—reportedly, it happened to be an area of great interest to the man who once revolutionized Silicon Valley.

Of all the advances in wearables, a no-prick diabetes sensor capable of alerting telemedicine physicians when sugar levels reach an unhealthy number could be the greatest indicator to date. This is due to the serious conditions associated with diabetes. The Mayo Clinic states this malady contributes to cardiovascular disease, neuropathy, kidney harm, eye damage, even Alzheimer's disease and dementia.[28] The tale of how diabetes almost took the life of one coauthor's friend/client demonstrates the power a no-prick diabetes monitoring wearable can have for someone susceptible to this condition.

Steve Bagley is a grandfather and retiree after a long career in Christian ministry and counseling. He coauthored *Never Alone: A Man's Companion Guide to Grief* with Michael Ashley.[29] Little did the former know that a strawberry milkshake of all things would present a terrifying danger to his health. Soon after completing the book, Steve was at lunch with Michael celebrating.

But before we get into what happened, it should be noted, Steve had tried to manage prediabetes for a decade with varying success. The milkshake he had with Michael on a Friday sent his blood glucose level skyrocketing, but he had no idea he was in trouble. He stumbled through the weekend getting fuzzier and fuzzier. Finally, on Monday he focused all his energy on attending a scheduled diabetes test, which he went to despite feeling sick and disoriented. His physician, Dr. Ali, planned to review the results and then contact Steve on Tuesday to let him know how his blood glucose was looking.

The fact that Dr. Ali was suffering from insomnia Monday night is what saved Steve's life. As it happens, the good doctor called Steve at 1:00 a.m. to alert Steve about an anomaly he happened to catch in the wee hours. "Your blood sugar came back at 515—a dangerously high figure." Dr. Ali told Steve to call 911 and get an ambulance to his house immediately. A stubbornly good-natured man—even when not disoriented—Steve eventually drove himself to the ER at 4:00 a.m. Here, doctors and nurses worked feverishly to bring his blood sugar under control, saving him from a diabetic coma. Or death.

Steve got lucky because his doctor couldn't sleep that night. It could have gone another way. Now, how might this story have played out with Apple's no-prick technology combined with telemedicine? Steve would be wearing his Apple Watch, and his telemedicine provider would proactively alert spikes to Steve's blood sugar. When the milkshake in question sent Steve into a downward spiral, a telemedicine physician not unlike Dr. Ali would contact him to coordinate a fast response—instead of the legacy healthcare system's approach of relying on a disoriented senior understanding his symptoms *and* seeking care.

The bottom line?

This wearable, and those described previously, offer to transform people—especially seniors—from being passive patients into active participants in their own healthcare. What we're describing is the shift of telemedicine from being an urgent care service providing help in times of illness and distress into offering a primary care relationship for patients. This shift is made possible by the development of interconnected care, whereby stakeholders, including the patient and their physician, receive real-time data *together*—and can make wise health decisions based on it. The ability to measure so many disparate factors reliably, and in real time, will allow telemedicine physicians to create better health outcomes, all while saving time by cutting out needless travel and waiting.

As we've seen, this idea isn't science fiction. It's not even particularly speculative. A *New York Times* piece from January 2023 explains how wearables and real-time data are revolutionizing healthcare *today*.[30] Telemedicine will be one more factor enabling tech to reach its true potential.

WHEN HOME IS BETTER THAN HOSPITAL

The *Times* also documents the technology driving the future of medicine in an article titled, "Your Next Hospital Bed Might Be at Home," by physician and Columbia University professor Helen Ouyang.[31] Dr. Ouyang's piece explains the hospital-at-home model gaining traction. Marquee healthcare organizations like Kaiser Permanente are investing in this new approach. It allows patients to get better where they feel most comfortable instead of in a hospital. As just one positive outcome, hospital beds are freed up for ICU units and other services truly requiring hospital care.

Still, the legacy healthcare approach to hospital-at-home is not without challenges. For one thing, it flips the inefficiency of the legacy system, putting the onus on providers. Instead of patients commuting to appointments, doctors and nurses must travel around, spending time in transit instead of helping patients lead healthier lives. In our view, *both* parties should enjoy the benefits of hospital-at-home by delivering the majority of care via telemedicine.

As the article also explains, real-time data telemetry and wearable monitors are *already* where they need to be for this to work. Consider Dr. Ouyang's description of 87-year-old dementia patient Rita Nelson. She was treated using the hospital-at-home philosophy while living with her niece, Susan Johnson. The piece describes the interplay between Johnson, Nurse Valerie Frazier, and experts acting as telemedicine providers.

> A few minutes later, the tablet and Frazier's phone started ringing: Did Nelson fall down? Because Frazier had folded the Biofourmis patch into her pocket, an alert had been sent out. Three people immediately checked in: the nurse practitioner, a Biofourmis nurse and the nurse coordinator for the trial.
>
> This oversight continued throughout the night.

The piece goes on to describe how the close monitoring, augmented by the devices (the phone, tablet, and the Biofourmis patch), provided immense peace of mind. Nelson's heart rate had dropped, but adequate alerts assured help.[32]

The patient received extraordinary care via the combination of wearables and telemedicine, all while enjoying the side benefits of living at home. Here, she ate hearty meals of her favorite foods and became active again after refusing to leave her bed or eat in the hospital. Symptoms like pressure sores on her feet disappeared, and her condition improved. The article ends with a description of the tremendous benefits of hospital-at-home on Rita's life.[33]

Undoubtedly, Rita Nelson's life improved thanks to the combination of getting her out of a hospital, putting her in a good family environment, and encouraging activity levels—all while monitoring her through breakthrough wearable tech, real-time data, and telemedicine. This uplifting story offers the future of telemedicine. It is a message of hope for a better, healthier America, and more positive outcomes for both patients and doctors.

Now that we know what's already possible today, it's time to go to the realm of science ~~fiction~~ fact. In Part III, we explore what tomorrow will soon offer us medically, starting with our minds.

PART III

TOMORROW

CHAPTER 9

Remote-Based Behavioral Health

It's March 6, 2027. Ramón Montoya should be happy. Bright and talented, he's turning 18 and graduating from high school in a few months. But the young man is stuck in a rut. He feels his life has no purpose. His grades have been slipping despite his obvious academic gifts. He also hasn't bothered filling out college applications though he once dreamed of becoming an engineer.

What Ramón doesn't know? His life will take quite a turn next month.

But first, Ramón is a second-generation American living in Brooklyn. His grandfather moved to the Big Apple from Iquitos, Peru, in the Amazon rainforest. Since then, his family has prospered considerably. And although Brazil is often the first thing that comes to mind when we think of the Amazon, the rainforest actually covers 60 percent of *Peru's* land.[1]

Ramón's ancestors hail from there. He knows if he looked back far enough, he would find he is, in fact, a descendant of the jungle. But Ramón doesn't dwell much on the subject. Family history bores the teen. Like many youngsters, he's more interested in playing video games with friends.

Video games offer Ramón an escape from life's drudgery, but they aren't a depression treatment. For that, he sees a therapist weekly using a telehealth service to speak from the privacy of his own room. Also, he self-medicates, regularly smoking marijuana and drinking to excess. He's had some brushes with the law as a result, not to mention trouble in school.

He hopes to have fun at his upcoming birthday, not understanding just how important it will be to his future. Filled with family members, many he hasn't seen in years, the party draws Ramón out of his shell. It's a joyous occasion. Four generations attend. Conversant in Spanish but not fluent, Ramón can't always follow his older relatives' friendly banter. Still, he has a great time enjoying Peruvian favorites like *ceviche* and his grandma's famous *ají de gallina*.

After the cake is cut, Ramón receives presents, mostly cash credit for his PlayStation. He notices his grandfather holds an envelope but hasn't handed it over, making Ramón curious about what it might be. At some point, most of the family filters out of the house, leaving only Ramón, his parents, and his siblings, plus his grandfather still holding the mysterious envelope.

Ramón looks into the old man's eyes. "*Abuelito*, what's in there? You thinking about keeping my birthday gift for yourself?"

His grandfather smiles. "What's in this envelope, I don't need. Ramón, I love you, and I want to give you a special present. I know you're struggling. My gift is something that's helped members of this family find their way for generations. I hope it helps you too."

Ramón is confused. "What are you talking about?"

Taking the envelope, he opens it to find not a card stuffed with cash, but a printed paper indicating his grandfather has covered all expenses for Ramón to meet with a shamanic practitioner based in his ancestral homeland.

The teen looks up in disbelief. "Um. You want me to see a witch doctor?"

Ramón's grandfather chuckles. So do his other nearby relatives. "I know. It sounds crazy. But a shaman helped me find my life's direction. I only came to this country because of what I learned about myself—with a shaman's help. And it helped your dad too."

Ramón turns to his father. "*You*? The most strait-laced guy in Brooklyn. You took a trip with a shaman?"

His dad just grins. "I needed to know my place so I got help, just like people from our culture have for thousands of years. Now it's your turn."

Still, Ramón isn't sold. He's freaked out. "Yo, I'm *not* going to the Peruvian jungle to drink some crazy tea and get high with strangers. Forget it."

"You don't go *anywhere*. We found a shaman on the same telehealth app you use to see a therapist. Grandpa's footing the bill. No travel involved."

"No *physical* travel," his grandfather adds, sharing a knowing glance.

Days pass and Ramón's reluctance wanes a bit.

He agrees to have the first of several sessions with a telemedicine shaman despite misgivings. He books a session for three days out. Just as he would for any therapy session, Ramón goes to his room and opens the app the day of the meeting. He doesn't know what to expect, but the young man who greets him on the other side of the screen sure isn't it. The person he sees doesn't look at all like a traditional healer. His English is also polished, with only a small trace of an accent.

"*Hola*, my name is Carlos," the young man begins. "I'm glad to start you on your journey."

"Uh, you don't look like . . . like what I was thinking."

Carlos laughs. "I'm a *shaman in training*. My grandfather is who you will work with. You can think of me as his translator and his tech support team—all rolled into one."

Ramón thinks it all too strange to be true. "So, are you, like, sitting in some building on Long Island?"

Carlos does appear to be in an office setting, but he turns his camera toward a window displaying a lush forest. "No, I live and work with my grandfather here. We're as deep into the bush as you can be and still get a decent internet connection."

Ramón continues to be skeptical. "And the ayahuasca you want me to drink . . . does that come from some factory farm in Ohio?"

Carlos takes this in stride too. "Not at all. The plants comprising the brew have been cultivated by my hands, my father's hands, and his father's hands, just as they have been for centuries. Everything comes from the source."

Ramón lowers his defenses. He asks for an explanation of the process. He soon learns he will be expected to be on a special diet for weeks. This is to "purify" his body. Ramón shall also abstain from all drugs and alcohol. Even coffee. After that? He is to take part in a ceremony led by Carlos's grandfather, the shaman. The latter will assist the teen on his spiritual journey, interpret his experiences, and enable integration when it's over.

"But there is a modern twist," Carlos adds. "In one key way we integrate a Western approach. Throughout it all, we will be monitoring your vital signs using a wearable directly connected to the telemedicine service."

"You mean a Fitbit?"

"Something like that."

After a few more questions, Ramón closes the session out. He thinks about what he is to undergo for the next few days until a box arrives on his doorstep. Inside, it includes everything he will need for his medicinal trip, including detailed instructions on brewing the ayahuasca tea included in carefully sealed packages marked as having been filled in Peru. Now committed to the process, he keeps himself busy to avoid eating fast food, smoking weed, and drinking alcohol—all no-no's on Carlos's preparation list.

In the next few days Ramón clears his head and his body. He also shifts his perspective. He begins to feel real excitement about his upcoming experience. Anticipation he hasn't known in years builds within him. In his free time, he reads—and rereads—instructions for the ceremony, wondering just what it will entail. He comes across a report in *Healthline* that stresses that those taking ayahuasca "need to be looked after carefully, as an Ayahuasca trip leads to an altered state of consciousness that lasts for many hours."[2]

Another description of the process posted on the site mindbodygreen.com can't help but freak Ramón out: "You'll probably vomit profusely, but purge buckets will be provided." Still, he's somewhat relieved, and intrigued, to learn of possible psychological benefits to the experience. From the same site: "The experience will be ineffable, beyond language, and you will likely find that trying to put it into words after the ceremony has ended will be daunting if not impossible. 'Ten years of therapy downloaded in a night,' seems to be a fairly universal analogy to convey the possible take-away from a ceremony."[3]

Ramón brings his concerns to his family, but both his father and his grandfather are quick to assure him it won't be as bad as it sounds. "I barely puked at all when I did it," the latter said. "Yes, it's intense, but I know you, and you can take it."

Nearly a month after his birthday, it's time. On the day of the ceremony, Ramón slips the wearable monitor onto his wrist and clicks to join the call on his tablet, his heart racing. Carlos's beatific face greets him. He stands beside an older man with a lined face and wispy gray hair. "Ramón, welcome! Allow me to introduce my grandfather Cleofe. He is our honored shaman, or as we call him, *Ayahuasquero*. You ready to learn what the vine of the soul has to show you?"

Tamping down fear, the teen nods, greeting the elderly healer with respect. He says something in a language Ramón doesn't understand, but Carlos quickly translates. "My grandfather says he can tell you're ready. He will now start the ceremony as you brew your tea."

Carlos triggers the telemedicine app to play ayahuasca *icaros*, special songs to carry the ceremony's energy, directing it in particular directions. At the same time, his grandfather chants. Carefully following the instructions in his package, Ramón prepares the tea, pouring himself a cup.

The old man speaks again, and once more, Carlos translates. "Drink deeply now, and then open your senses. Listen to the music. Concentrate on what you require help most with in this life."

Ramón follows the instructions. He gulps down the bitter, nasty brew. He listens to the music and the growing chanting with his eyes closed. Concentrating his mind, he centers on the question that has troubled him in recent days: *Should I pursue my dream of becoming an engineer or just forget it and go to work right now for my dad?*

As minutes roll by, Ramón worries he's done something wrong. Nothing is happening. *Did I mess up? Is this shaman a charlatan?* But when he opens his eyes to ask Carlos, his jaw drops instead. He isn't in his room anymore. He's in the rainforest. Ramón experiences several different visions in quick succession. He witnesses three men who appear to exist outside of time. They speak to him in an alien language he somehow understands. They tell him they are his relatives. Their message is clear: *You are one of us. We are proud of you. And you* are *capable.*

After the men leave, Ramón encounters a frightening jaguar with glowing red eyes. Somehow, he doesn't fear the beast. Anyway, it doesn't seem interested in attacking him. It shows Ramón a path through an impenetrable forest. Eventually these fade away, and Ramón is back in his room.

Carlos makes eye contact with the teen now bathed in sweat. To his astonishment, the bucket beneath Ramón is filled with his own vomit.

"Welcome back! You've been gone for several hours. Let's talk about what you experienced and what it means for your life."

With Carlos translating, Ramón explains to the shaman how he met his ancestors and a spirit animal. The shaman interprets his visions, explaining how the jaguar appearing to him meant the message was about the present, not the future, and that the insight was that he should act with confidence.

Carlos then asks, "So what'll you do with this information?"

Still shaky, Ramón is already on his feet. "I have some college applications to fill out."

Although he didn't share his personal experiences with his father or grandfather, both saw changes in Ramón. They noticed he wasn't smoking pot and had no interest in video games. Ramón seemed to have a new purpose. A few months later, they celebrated his acceptance to UC, Berkeley and the start of his life's journey, discovered in much the same way their own was, following the venerable centuries-old traditions of their culture.

EXPANDING THE UNIVERSE OF TREATMENT OPTIONS

Ramón's tale—unique as it is—contains a critical point to our discussion. The shaman-guided ceremony, so integral to his family's tradition, occurred via the same remote service his (Western) therapist already used to work with the teen. Following the six pillars of telemedicine we have established, in the future, a much wider range of treatments will undoubtedly be available for patients seeking such desired health outcomes.

Here's one example. Based on QuickMD's many past successes with rapidly expanding TeleMAT treatments to underserved areas, it isn't hard to imagine expanding the reach of a traditional Chinese medicine (TCM) practitioner.[4] This person could be located in San Francisco's

Chinatown yet treat patients as far away as Nebraska or using telemedicine in real time. Even so, we do expect some alternative treatments like chiropractic adjustments and acupuncture to require the human touch until advanced robotics are available at a consumer level. But in the meantime? Novel experiences like Ramón's are closer to current-day reality than one may think.

Although many exciting breakthroughs may be had upon applying telemedicine to alternative care, one source of inspiration for practitioners is the rapid pace of advancement to the mental health field. In many respects, behavioral care leads the charge to embrace telemedicine. We now explore how the mental health of so many Americans, particularly our young and vulnerable populations, are being positively affected by the embrace of bleeding-edge technology.

MEETING TEENS WHERE THEY'RE MOST COMFORTABLE

It is no exaggeration to suggest the typical young person is glued to their smartphone. According to a Pew Research survey published in 2022, about half of Americans in this demographic admit they are on their device "almost constantly." Most of the remaining participants confess they are on it several times a day, with just 3 percent saying they check in once every 24 hours.[5]

If you're curious what they're doing on their phones, they mostly engage with apps like YouTube, TikTok, Instagram, and Snapchat. What do all of those platforms have in common? They are primarily platforms for video and images. Meanwhile, years of social media exposure from a young age have trained teens to communicate with others through screens, making telehealth particularly useful in treating so many mental and behavioral concerns of this age group.

Critics may claim the trend of young people favoring their phone and other devices for communication—over in-person interactions—is a by-product of the COVID-19 pandemic. They say things will snap back to "normal" someday. This argument collapses when we examine data on the subject from before 2020. Long before lockdowns, teens already relied on tech to communicate with the outside world. *Time* reported in 2018 that two-thirds of surveyed young Americans prefer to communicate with friends via texting, video chat, and social media, while just a third preferred in-person meetings. According to survey administrator Common Sense Media, this is a dramatic change from 2012, when 49 percent of teenagers preferred in-person meetings with friends.[6]

As is well documented by now, American teens struggled with mental health problems during the pandemic. The CDC reported in 2022 that 37 percent of high schoolers reported poor mental health, and 44 percent felt persistently sad or hopeless.[7] As a result, some enterprising health companies, especially agile start-ups, jumped into the fray to combat mental health issues among teens and children in much the same way QuickMD has leapt into the battle against the opioid epidemic.

One such company is Brightline.

HOW BRIGHTLINE MAKES A POSITIVE IMPACT

Brightline bills itself as offering "virtual behavioral health coaching and therapy for families with kids ages 0 to 17 years old. Brightline's expert team of coaches, therapists, and prescribers offers live sessions for your child with no long waitlists. Coaching programs are also available for parents and caregivers." Offering behavioral services to families, Brightline is also a pioneer in working with employers to offer health services to employees as a benefit.[8]

From the patient perspective, Brightline offers an interesting mix of care designed to help children and families facing different issues.

Most importantly, its coaches, therapists, and physicians meet teens and children where they are most comfortable—on their devices. According to one recent article in the *World Journal of Psychiatry*, 85 percent of parents who used telehealth to treat their child's behavioral and mental health issues said their child *benefited from that care*.[9]

Brightline's embrace of tech has led it to expand to all 50 states. The first level of care concerns coaching based on cognitive behavior therapy (CBT), which the Mayo Clinic reports is for helping patients "become aware of inaccurate or negative thinking so you can view challenging situations more clearly and respond to them in a more effective way."[10] In Brightline's view, effective training for children, teens, and families can help overcome behavioral issues, like tantrums or anxiety. These coaching sessions typically run 30 minutes as the "first line of defense" in the company's lineup.

Along with such coaching, Brightline offers 55-minute-long sessions with licensed therapists and psychologists. ADHD, depression, and anxiety are commonly treated at this level. When needed, the company can provide medication support at an additional cost. Most importantly, Brightline can demonstrate effective results for its novel type of care.

According to the company's outcome summary on disruptive behaviors, 80 percent of parents whose kids attended coaching or therapy through Brightline reported significant improvements. When it comes to anxiety, Brightline's data shows 70 percent of parents report clinical progress, with 100 percent of parents who completed the company's pediatric anxiety treatment plan reporting some degree of success.[11] And patients suffering from depression also enjoyed impressive results. Brightline's published results demonstrate that 80 percent of patients improved their score, according to the outcomes scale developed by the National Institutes of Health (NIH).[12]

Brightline also makes a convincing case to employers as to how its service can empower businesses to run better. Just as QuickMD patients don't need to take a day off work to visit a doctor, Brightline's customers are more productive when they aren't overwhelmed with their children's mental health. Brightline's proposition and other companies like it is simple: happier families make for more productive workers.

Despite such a pitch to corporations, Brightline's focus stays firmly on young patients and the families supporting them. Founder and CEO Naomi Allen published an explanation of telehealth benefits for behavioral care in *Fast Company*. Here, you'll recognize the six telemedicine pillars woven into her argument: "Virtual care models are proven to improve outcomes for common challenges among children and teens, such as depression, ADHD, and anxiety." With virtual care, "more families can find the care they need, which might not have been accessible before due to distance, time restraints, or other barriers." It can be especially important in regions that lack resources for children's behavioral health and places with struggling LBGTQ+ youth.[13]

Clearly, Brightline's approach offers to vastly expand treatment options for families seeking optimal care for children. Happily, they aren't alone in witnessing telemedicine's benefits in the treatment of behavioral health. To learn more, we sat down to discuss this subject with trailblazing psychiatrist and thought leader Dr. Kenneth C. Nash.

TELEHEALTH IS MAKING A DIFFERENCE AT THE UNIVERSITY OF PITTSBURGH

Dr. Ken Nash has an admirable resume and an even more impressive ability to help his patients, especially youngsters, achieve desired mental health outcomes. Practicing at the University of Pittsburgh Department of Psychiatry, he also serves as professor and vice chair for clinical affairs for the Department of Psychiatry. The department is one of the largest recipients of National Institutes of Health funding for psychiatric research. In his role as chief of clinical services, Dr. Nash oversees more than two hundred psychiatric members of the UPMC Presbyterian medical staff and oversees a vast behavioral health network.

Beyond his academic duties and his psychiatry practice, Dr. Nash works as chief of clinical services at UPMC Western Psychiatric Hospital. Extending his commitment to the mental health of young people, he serves as the co-principal investigator for the Youth and Family Training Institute (YFTI). This is dedicated to providing High Fidelity Wraparound (HFW) care to youngsters throughout Pennsylvania. Of all Dr. Nash's many hats, this last one is particularly interesting because of the impact telemedicine can make on HFW services.

Dr. Nash's organization defines HFW as "a team-based, collaborative process for developing and implementing individualized plans for youth with complex behavioral health and/or other challenges, and their families."[14] The YFTI focuses its efforts on training service providers to coordinate treatment through four phases—engagement, planning, implementation, and transition. In practice, HFW is delivered via a combination of compassionate coaches. These are skill-based teachers and facilitators who develop plans to achieve positive outcomes. They are also avid family support partners that directly support patients' family members and youth support partners—typically people under age 25 who provide direct support to young patients.

With many moving parts and a large team interacting with youth in various capacities on a regular basis, telemedicine's effective usage can reduce the massive logistics needed to offer a life-changing care standard—especially for those in crisis. To learn more about cutting-edge applications to psychiatry and mental health treatment, we sat down with Dr. Nash in between a patient session and, ironically, a training on the University of Pittsburgh's latest telemedicine system.

When asked about his general opinion of this emerging field, Dr. Nash is overwhelmingly positive. "I love telehealth. My first telehealth visit was a psychiatry medication evaluation in the late 90s. We've come a long way from those days! These days, I view it as another modality to meet my patients. It has been around for some time, but obviously kicked into high gear during the pandemic. The tech was already there to support our work, but the changes we've seen concern adapting regulations and so many insurance payers now willing to reimburse for telemedicine. Certainly, I'm thrilled by the possibilities of telehealth. For one thing, we saw its successes in our own data and patient responses when we went fully remote during the pandemic. Now, in the post-pandemic period, we seek a balance, determining what can be better done with telehealth, and which is more appropriately handled in person. Each practitioner I work with is exploring what is best for the patient and provider."

Dr. Nash continues, "Telehealth is here to stay. The great results we've seen, both from practitioners and psychiatrists, are too strong. Too compelling. I support every method to connect patients to mental health providers, whether it's telehealth or the ability to message outside of appointments with an app."

We asked Dr. Nash to expand on striking the balance between in-person visits and telehealth sessions. Just what goes into finding that equilibrium he described? He explains, "It comes down to a combination of what the patient responds best to and assessing the appropriate approach. For example, I don't see myself performing surgery via telehealth. On the other hand, I've been able to provide therapy sessions to patients that have been extremely effective—especially patients who have struggled with in-person sessions."

Dr. Nash stresses that telehealth isn't new to his field but is finally a realistic treatment option. "Remote care provides a great environment for improved mental health outcomes. For years, we knew it was effective, and we knew patients liked it—but regulations and payers held us back. We performed one local study that always sticks with me—the results showed how young people prefer telehealth to in-person visits. Our retention rate was significantly higher in certain populations based on this satisfaction. At the end of the day, patient preference, clinical issues, and workforce availability often align to make telehealth an ideal solution."

When asked why he thought young people scored telemedicine so highly on the quality survey, Dr Nash explained it this way, "The younger a person is, the likelier they are to find telehealth acceptable. That goes for patients and providers. Older folks tend to be less receptive, yet even the oldest people in each category typically don't push back against telehealth once they try it. Any reluctance tends to come from payers and regulatory bodies."

He continued, "I also think young people are especially more comfortable connecting to physicians, therapists, and psychiatrists the same way they connect to other things in their life—via their smartphones and other devices. Their attitude is, 'I get everything through my phone, why shouldn't I get healthcare the same way?' In fact, I've treated young people who say their best friend is someone they've met online, someone who lives in another state. If you can make close friendships remotely, you can also form an effective treatment relationship online. Critically, I tend to see patients engaged in their own care. They are choosing to improve their mental health through telehealth instead of being forced into an uncomfortable in-person clinical environment."

We next asked Dr. Nash for his views on how telehealth can help mental health professionals integrate with primary care practices.

"Therapists and psychiatrists are finding considerable value to telehealth in how it integrates. Picture a therapist who works across a primary care practice. If that practice has five different locations, the therapist has two options—create a complicated schedule of hours between locations or remove the logistical nightmare by utilizing telemedicine. The result is going to be a more productive therapist *and* more patients receiving quality care."

Dr. Nash says internal data backs up telehealth benefits. "Our remote visits enjoy a higher show rate than in-person visits. In other words, a telehealth patient is likelier to make an appointment than an in-person patient. The fact they don't have to fight traffic and/or deal with life's other complexities to get here contributes to that, but I think it's also because healthcare consumers are opting to be more involved in their own treatment."

There are major advancements to be made in telehealth, according to Nash. This is especially true as concerns the team-based approach with High Fidelity Wraparound treatment of at-risk young people. "There's an attitude that telehealth is about meeting the 'doctor in charge' for an appointment. I believe as data gets better and new standards are created, telehealth will expand in HFW with a more diverse team participating in sessions. Our patients are young people with complex mental health and behavioral challenges. The more we can get their peer support and other non-licensed team members involved, instead of just their primary caregivers, the better the outcome is likely to be."

Dr. Nash believes that teleconsults, or doctors using telehealth services to speak to other doctors, can also help primary care physicians become more proactive and less reactive going forward. He explained how the process could benefit doctors: "Let's say a primary care physician is worried about obesity in a patient. Perhaps they can't afford a dietitian onsite to meet with patients who would benefit from dietary improvements. Teleconsults could open the door to better health outcomes for these patients if their primary care physician can work with a specialist in real time to create a plan of action. Naturally, this type of teleconsult creates its own staffing issues, but it still gives the primary care doctor the ability to diversify to meet patient needs."

Wearables play their own vital role in driving telehealth's future success. As Dr. Nash explains, "We're seeing more patients that have data at their fingertips from such devices, and it's a huge benefit. The best area now is sleep tracking. If you ask me how I slept last night, my answer may be poorly correlated to actual data from my Oura Ring. Of course, we would never say to a patient, 'Hey, how's your blood pressure doing?' or 'How's your pulse today?' but somehow, for sleep—something incredibly important to our mental and physical health—we've been happy to accept basic opinions based on tangential information, like a loud sound waking you up at 2:00 a.m."

He continued, "But I think wearables also empower patients to learn about their own health and to affect it accordingly. For example, I've learned that if I eat late at night, the amount of deep sleep I get after that goes down. Because I have access to that data, I can make better choices for my own health. I couldn't do that without the Oura Ring I wear nightly."

Confidentiality will always be a mental health concern, something Dr. Nash remains mindful of. "As a psychiatrist, I'm dealing with data far more sensitive, far more personal than heart rates. That makes me as mindful, if not more, of privacy concerns than practically anyone else in the medical field. Given that concern, wearables offer advantages to continuous monitoring. For me, it boils down to being able to get a truer picture of what's going on with my patients so I can help them to the fullest extent of my abilities."

We asked Dr. Nash to explain more—what a wearable can tell him that his patient can't. He elaborated, "A lot of patients will tell me what's going on in their lives. They're reporting what happened in the last month, but in reality, it could be what they've felt in the *last hour*. I don't live with my patients, obviously. I see them once every few weeks. Yet when there's a source of data beyond a patient's own report, I now have a better gauge on how things are actually progressing. I get that true picture of the month without the subjectivity of the patient's answer being impacted by the most recent events."

He continued, "Although I can't share a patient example of this phenomenon with you, I can describe one from my own life. In August, I suffered a ruptured disc in my back. Over the course of several months, you could see how the injury impacted my sleep—using recorded data. At first it disrupted my deep sleep. But that improved steadily over several months. Now I'm sleeping normally again. But if you asked me at any point how I was sleeping, I probably would have answered 'awful.' Once I had data to see the true picture, my perception changed. Put simply, sleep data gave me valuable quantifiable information. Insights into my health provided by the wearable were invaluable, and I'm seeing the same phenomenon with my own patients."

Dr. Nash concluded the interview by explaining how he's gratified to see so many primary care physicians catching up to their mental health peers. "Behavioral health has had an easier time realizing telemedicine's advantages because our specialty lends itself more to the adoption of new technology. For some time, we've been helping patients with phobias confront their fears in a safe virtual reality environment. Now it's a positive for American healthcare to see other areas like urgent care, MAT for addiction, and medically supervised weight loss catching up. At the end of the day, positive patient health outcomes are what really matters, and telehealth is a wonderful tool to improve them."

TECH IS ALWAYS EVOLVING

As we have seen, telemedicine benefits greatly from innovations, whether it is the vast improvement in video quality afforded by the latest generation of smartphones or the internet infrastructure providing more reliable connectivity. The field will continue progressing to incorporate new advancements to benefit more patients. But the latest emerging field? AI.

Artificial intelligence is *already* playing a role in mental health treatment. And it will continue to do so. Just a few years before the COVID pandemic, an AI chatbot named rAInbow launched to help victims of domestic abuse in emerging countries understand their rights and how they can seek help.[15] Importantly, this app doesn't replace a human therapist or any number of other humans who may help a victim of domestic abuse, but it does serve as another piece in the treatment puzzle. Only time will tell if AI will continue to play an important role in expanding the ability of telemedicine to make patients healthier. Our guess? AI's best days are ahead of us when it comes to intelligently and compassionately treating us humans.

Now it's time to shift gears to cover a different future-related subject. We will assess what emerging telehealth policies and laws will mean for business, especially investors, now that we are out of the COVID-19 pandemic crisis.

CHAPTER 10

Will Government Throw a Wrench in Telehealth?

Jared Sheehan opens his eyes 15 seconds before his alarm goes off. Ever since he started wearing an Oura Ring sleep tracker to bed, he's been getting the best sleep of his life, despite the heavy weight of being the head of operations for QuickMD—and coauthor of the book in your hands. He knows his phone will soon burst with notifications from doctors, partner organizations, and all sorts of other people wanting his time. Even so, he forces himself not to check his email and social updates until after his first cup of coffee.

He knows he is in for a busy day, but Jared repeats his usual daily mantra: "It's a good problem to have."

Returning to the sleep tracker, it was one of his doctor's suggestions under the concierge medical program offered by his own company. It feels funny logging into the QuickMD app as a patient instead of as an employer, but it has produced wonders for his health and given him a new perspective on operations. His doctor also suggested modifications to Jared's diet, including healthier breakfast fare, which he eats as he wades through messages.

Today is an especially busy day because his cofounders are offline. Dr. Omer is presenting at a symposium in Europe, speaking to a diverse audience of physicians and healthcare investors about QuickMD's rapid U.S. growth and the innovative ways the company has found new applications for telemedicine, from urgent care and opioid addiction to weight loss and concierge care. He is also planting seeds for a potential expansion of QuickMD overseas.

The third cofounder, Chris Rovin, is taking his first vacation in three years. He's off to Singapore to taste all of the delectable exotic foods he can with limited Wi-Fi access, definitely a first for yet another avowed workaholic. Of course Jared knows that since he isn't a doctor he won't be making medical decisions for Dr. Omer, but he will be filling Chris's shoes by managing QuickMD's roster of physicians scattered around the country. Jared is especially happy for Chris to take time off as he looks forward to his own planned vacation soon. The extra work makes Jared's busy day even more hectic, but for the second time today, he tells himself: "It's a good problem to have."

The first message Jared gets is from a person we'll call Dr. James. Noticing the urgent flag, he's reminded how good Chris is with managing physicians and hopes he doesn't end up causing his friend and cofounder unnecessary headaches. Dr. James's urgent message concerns two doctors he referred to QuickMD as potential hires. He's worried that after two days, neither individual has heard from their organization.

Reading the email makes Jared reflect back on Dr. James's own introduction to QuickMD. It was truly a case of "third time's the charm." A family doctor, he previously enjoyed—or suffered—from a busy practice depending on your perspective. One of his close colleagues joined the telemedicine start-up and implored him to give it a shot.

At first Dr. James didn't want to talk to Dr. Omer about the opportunity. "Telehealth isn't for me. It's a passing fad, not a career." Even when a second colleague joined QuickMD and approached him independently,

Dr. James had the same answer. Only a third discussion—with both his close friends at once—changed his mind. What made a stubborn doctor set in his ways consider making the professional leap? The enhanced life quality his colleagues were enjoying.

Dr. James knew as soon as he met his colleagues for lunch that they had indeed found amazing new careers. They looked rested, happy, and energized by the difference they were making fighting the opioid epidemic. Over sushi rolls and sake, they told their former coworker about patient success stories. They also related how much they enjoyed a new work-life balance that, as one put it, "actually involves balance, instead of all career and no life."

This conversation struck a chord with Dr. James, especially because his complex work schedule left him precious little time with his sick father. After several weeks of discussions, Dr. James joined QuickMD, first on a part-time basis and then becoming a full-time practitioner. He has since excelled in telehealth, earning rave reviews from his many patients.

Even better, he also experienced a complete shift in his work-life balance. These days, instead of getting to see his dad once every few weeks—often at the rest home while the latter is sleeping—he visits him *daily*. He blocks off his schedule from 2:00 to 4:00 p.m. to spend an hour with his father when he's most alert. "I don't have kids," he said. "But I understand the pain my coworkers felt not being there for theirs because I wasn't there for my dad. All that changed when I entered telemedicine."

His success and the ensuing transformation of his personal life turned Dr. James into a telehealth proponent. He's not alone. Jared knows other QuickMD physicians who similarly have become evangelists. They get so much from helping patients through their toughest times while not sacrificing their own lives. It's no surprise they want to bring this opportunity to their peers. Having identified additional prospects, Dr. James was nervous his new employer still hadn't contacted them.

Jared writes him an email explaining how several of those on the leadership team are out of the office and that referrals are coming in so fast QuickMD is struggling to keep up. After thanking the doctor for his great work and promising to contact the prospects soon, Jared sends his message off. Afterward, he can't help reflecting on how there are now so many doctors referring potential hires they can afford to scale back job advertisements in certain states.

Again, he repeats his mantra of the day: "It's a good problem to have!"

The next urgent matter concerns new hires. A month ago, QuickMD's advanced data analysis systems detected a developing opioid hotspot in Mississippi. While the legacy healthcare system might take years to establish strong brick-and-mortar infrastructure for such underserved communities, QuickMD jumped into action immediately. A call went out to the growing team of physicians seeking new doctors within the state. The program, much like employee referral incentives offered at other corporations, offers a bonus for every hired doctor to serve this demographic.

Dr. Francesca Martinez, who lives in nearby Louisiana, proved to be a superstar recruiter based on her relationships across the border in nearby Mississippi. In fact, she referred three doctors who were soon hired on and put into service treating opioid addicts using the lifesaving TeleMAT technique. Now she wishes to be compensated for her efforts. Dr. Martinez, like most physicians in the legacy healthcare system, knows reimbursement can be slow. She's used to duking it out with insurance carriers. Still, she kept a friendly tone in her note to QuickMD asking when she can expect her referral bonus.

For Jared, this is an easier problem to tackle than the last message. He contacts accounting and asks them to include the money in her next paycheck. Then he lets Dr. Martinez know when to expect payment without mentioning that the hiccup occurred because the team is growing so fast. As if he's talking to his fellow cofounders, Jared tells the empty room, "If we're saving lives faster than our accounting department can move, it's another good problem to have."

But Jared's string of *good* problems is about to end.

Urgent messages out of the way, Jared grabs lunch and prepares for his first scheduled meeting. He is to chat with an investment bank VP who has expressed interest in investing in QuickMD. Like any start-up that scaled fast, Jared and his cofounders recognize they have a winning formula. Still, outside investment could help them save more lives and rapidly improve patient outcomes on a wider scale.

Jared feels upbeat about the meeting, especially since he has promising stats to share. After exchanging pleasantries over Zoom, Jared launches into impressive facts about QuickMD. He describes its recent growth and high patient satisfaction scores. He also explains his team's ability to penetrate new geographic areas, using Mississippi as an example. Last, he mentions their intention to focus on other areas, like medication-assisted weight loss, and to embrace new tech in the wearables field.

Jared pauses here to gauge the VP's reaction.

It starts out well. She tells Jared, "This is all very impressive. You've built a strong business that's making a difference in people's lives. However, that isn't all that counts to investors. People like me need to know we will get a return on what we put in. And that requires a stable regulatory environment. Until the fallout from COVID is better understood, any company operating under the Public Health Emergency laws is un-investable."

Jared keeps his composure throughout the rest of the call.

Before it ends, he promises to stay in touch. Still, he can't help feeling shaken. A profitable business enjoying fantastic growth—so much so that he can't hire personnel fast enough—while achieving the altruistic goal of saving lives—is *un-investable*? He wants to call Dr. Omer and Chris to strategize but stops himself. He will just have to wait until everyone is back. (Meaning, they are online again. All internal employees work remotely.)

Moreover, for the first time today, Jared is forced to admit this is a *very bad problem to have*.

UNDERSTANDING THE RED TAPE IS CRUCIAL

Although parts of the tale you just read were changed to protect privacy, the downbeat ending is accurate. Regulatory uncertainty *is* preventing the investment community from putting big money into telemedicine—this despite its proven ability to respond to Americans' healthcare needs. Complex laws surrounding telehealth are acting as red tape, especially preventing underserved communities from getting needed help. This situation is challenging for patients regardless of their age and/or race, whether they live in urban, suburban, or rural locations.

From our vantage point, there's but one way to work through our legal dilemma, and that's to team up with top lawyers. In the telemedicine space, that means Foley & Lardner LLP. Chambers USA's *America's Leading Lawyers for Business* for 2020 through 2023 gives Foley's Telemedicine and Digital Health practice a glowing review. It describes the group as "the premier firm for telehealth counsel," as well as the "Dream Team" for telemedicine companies.[1]

To learn more about the regulatory challenges surrounding remote care and how companies like ours can (still) grow successfully while fighting for more commonsense telehealth regulations, we sat down with Foley partner Kyle Y. Faget. Calling Kyle a subject matter expert is an understatement. She's emerged as a trustworthy authority on telehealth regulations while also possessing a unique background as in-house counsel at precommercial and commercial stage companies. Kyle was also a Microsoft fellow at the University of Michigan law school, where she researched FDA regulations.

In short, Kyle is a leading light in efforts to create reasonable and effective telehealth regulations. To this end, she provided us with frank, insightful answers to questions swirling around telehealth—the same queries that leave investment bankers like the one Jared spoke to scared to commit.

SPECIAL REGISTRATION MAY BE THE KEY TO TELEMAT

We began by asking Kyle to explain why doctors who want to prescribe a controlled substance like TeleMAT medication Suboxone must see patients in-person and what solutions to that requirement may be possible. As she explains, "Under the Controlled Substances Act, an in-person visit is necessary to actually prescribe controlled substances. This goes back to the death of Ryan Haight and the law bearing his name. That was an era of telemedicine gone rogue. It meant anyone could go online and get any drug they wanted. The belief of regulators and legislators back then was that mandating an in-person visit may aid in preventing future tragic deaths or injuries. These laws date to a time before legitimate prescribers entered the mix."

On a positive note, she also explains how the situation may be shifting: "I'm hopeful the DEA will roll out a special telehealth registration, which is long overdue. During COVID-19, companies like QuickMD could prescribe controlled substances because the DEA waived the Ryan Haight provision. They had the authority to do so because of the public health emergency. What the DEA can't do is abandon the law wholesale. There must be a legislative fix to amend the

Ryan Haight Act and remove the in-office visit provision. Or we need to see the creation of a special telehealth registration. While I can't speak for the DEA, it would probably take the form of *credentialing* whereby the legitimacy of the prescriber is assessed and stamped by the agency."

She also adds context to how the government considers changes to law: "This all became particularly important during the pandemic because telemedicine emerged as a 'miracle cure.' It helped Americans get the healthcare they needed without coming into contact with others. As effective as telemedicine proved to be, it didn't change underlying ethical issues the DEA and other interested government parties worry about. Even now, they are trying to determine questions like, 'How do you sort out good actors from bad?' and 'Can this be done safely?' I hope this type of special registration is rolled out in the near future."[2]

WALKING THE EDGE OF THE TELEHEALTH CLIFF

Next, we asked Kyle to discuss the so-called telehealth cliff, one of the central concepts scaring investment bankers and venture capitalists alike.

Kyle explains, "The 'telehealth cliff' is related to waivers in the law. We have to back up a bit and consider those first. In the midst of the pandemic, waivers were put in place due to the public health emergency declared by the Secretary of Health and Human Services. These allowed agencies like the DEA to forgo requirements like those in the Ryan Haight Act for in-person visits to prescribe controlled substances. Other waivers were also granted. CMS relinquished a host of different requirements under what are called 1135 waivers, not just at the federal level. States waived many requirements affecting medical practice, too, like licensure requirements."

She elaborates on changes affecting the latter: "Typically speaking, Medicare was not provided in a patient's home. Government-compensated care occurred only in places where a statistical shortage of providers was present and/or rural geography was required for reimbursement. The kind of practitioners and the locations where telehealth visits could occur were limited. What happened during COVID is that many people were all of a sudden allowed to enjoy telehealth at home. This makes a big difference."

Even so, there were still important constraints to the new model. It wasn't a free-for-all. "The other thing is that the Office of Civil Rights, which oversees and enforces HIPAA compliance, said they would engage in enforcement *discretion*. In other words, people needn't engage in telehealth through a medium that would meet strict privacy requirements. Patients could FaceTime with a provider as an acceptable means. Before this, typically speaking, you would have to use a secure portal like you see with hospital systems for any real-time visual communication or telehealth visit. Other waivers at the state level included allowing clinicians to practice across state lines in many circumstances."

These waivers, Kyle explains, combine to form the basis of our now looming telehealth cliff. "Permissions were put in place at multiple government levels to facilitate telehealth during the public health emergency. When this ends, such waivers will go away without legislative action on all levels. The cliff comes into play when remote care companies that operated in the context of the waivers are suddenly asked to comply with pre-COVID regulations—unless they change."

Next, Kyle walks us through how telemedicine companies view the approaching cliff. "Organizations are thinking deeply about their operations, trying to work with their existing business models. Or updating them. If the latter is required, it will warrant extreme changes in many cases. Think about it. They are successfully doing business one way. Then overnight, waivers get rolled back, or OCR no longer takes the discretionary approach and HIPAA requires they go back to pre-COVID regulations. The question is, for example, if there is a 50-state virtual model for treating opioid addiction with controlled substances and a practice is now 100 percent virtual, how can you satisfy the Haight Act requirement for in-office visits? Clearly, there are no easy answers or magic wands right now."

THE POLITICS OF OUR TELEHEALTH CLIFF

The telehealth cliff has thorny political implications. Kyle shares her viewpoint on how the legacy practice of medicine is rooted in location. "It's been a largely local affair insofar as licensure boards dictate care standards. State governments may have laws and/or regulations that may say, for instance, that you must form a clinician/patient relationship through real-time audio and video communications. Only thereafter can you engage in asynchronous telehealth. That's pretty rare at this point, but just for example's sake, that might be something that is a law. Medical boards will then police and enforce such a requirement. Also, sometimes medical boards will have regulatory guidance to interpret regulations. A lot of that is really driven by state-level considerations. Still, it's important to understand it all when considering the idea of working around our telehealth cliff."

She continues, "There are state government and licensure boards, plus medical boards. There are also nursing boards based on the license. The result is various licensure boards overseeing practices. That's *one* side of the standard-of-care issue. Then there are payers. These can dictate what they will reimburse and how. Let's say we are discussing Medicare reimbursement. Asynchronous telemedicine may not meet the government's practice standards for reimbursement. The question then becomes: Can you legally engage in an asynchronous telehealth visit? *Sure*. But will you get paid for that visit? That depends on the payer and what it requires as a condition for reimbursement. Medicare has its own rules. Commercial payers have their own rules. You must look at what those contracts are to understand what those payers are requiring, and what it is that those payers will reimburse via telehealth and what they won't."

Kyle also believes there is a strong political element to this discussion. "It's very political, and I'll tell you why. Many states have commissioned a review of telehealth usage. (By the way, you see this at the federal level, too.) Pre-pandemic, the concern was always *overutilization*. Here's the idea. If we make healthcare super readily available, then Americans will want to talk to their doctor 27,000 times a week. Payers don't want to pay for that. There is absolute cause for concern here, particularly when the largest healthcare services payer in the United States is Medicare. Then, when you bundle in Medicaid, we're talking about a *huge* percentage of healthcare payments. Naturally, there's a vested interest in cost containment. When you make healthcare services so readily available, overutilization is the fear. There's also the question: What are the actual rates that should be reimbursed?"

Kyle goes on to explain: "We often discuss this in terms of payment parity. If you see a clinician in office, that visit, even if it takes the same amount of time, may or may not ultimately be paid at the same rate should the clinician spend the same amount of time with you online. The concept behind that is, 'Okay, Doctor. If you're using telehealth, isn't your overhead reduced? You needn't have a brick-and-mortar presence. It's cheaper for you to practice.' The reality is many providers engage in a *hybrid* practice. They still have overhead yet they're combining telehealth flexibility. Here's essentially the argument: 'Doctors, you've got reduced overhead. Therefore, why should we pay you the same amount we did when you were practicing in a brick-and-mortar location?'"

Of course, if you're a provider and you know you're going to get paid more to do something in office than via telehealth, incentives change. That's Kyle's view too: "Exactly. Those are points for contention. Before COVID, there wasn't enough telehealth to go around. It wasn't so ubiquitous like it is now that you could look at the situation analytically and say, 'Okay, now that telehealth is readily available, is there actually overutilization or not?' In the coming years we'll be able to answer that since we will have those numbers that didn't exist before."

HOW INSURANCE AFFECTS TELEMEDICINE

Next, Kyle discusses how private payers, most often insurers, will affect remote care moving forward. "Private payers decide what they will cover. During COVID, states legislated on this point. They said, 'If you're going to do business in our state, here's our minimum standard for payer requirements.' The big question, again, concerns parity: 'Are you, as a payer, going to cover that visit at the same rate as an office visit?' The result means differences in coverage. Suddenly, one person has access to care that may look different than their neighbor. That's huge. Whether you have United or Blue Cross, or Blue Shield, they all look different in terms of what they will or will not cover."

Combined with the government's reimbursement structure, private payer differences contribute to varying standards. Kyle adds, "There isn't a national rubric in America. Care standards are defined *locally*. Also, both coverage and reimbursement shift plan by plan. This is true for Medicare, as it's yet another healthcare plan with its own coverage limitations and determinations. You may even find there are coverage discrepancies across the United States. I don't know if this kind of geographic disparity exists in countries with national healthcare coverage, but I would expect to see much more uniformity in terms of what's covered and what isn't."

TELEMEDICINE'S FUTURE—SEEN THROUGH LAWYER EYES

Kyle expects even more shifts to the healthcare market soon. "As we come out of COVID and there's a change in the appetite for telehealth, we'll see a settling of laws and regulations. States will determine what they think is an acceptable care standard. Likewise, payers will decide what they want to cover and what they don't. The only way we'll see significant systemic changes over the next 15 to 20 years is if we opt for a national practice standard. Currently, state medical boards have a lot of power over medicine. I don't see them giving that up anytime soon."

She continues, "The best-case telemedicine scenario is if every state becomes a member of the interstate medical licensure compact, for example. This will allow clinicians who are fully licensed in one state to be readily licensed in all states across the U.S. That shift will create a much larger pool of potential clinicians businesses can tap into. If you pair this development with the DEA creating a telehealth registration, existing telehealth limits instead become limits of technology and medicine—rather than limits of government regulation."

UNDERSTANDING THE INVESTOR MINDSET

The protagonist of our story at the beginning of the chapter, Jared Sheehan, has been the tip of the QuickMD spear when it comes to working with investors. To round out this chapter's discussion, we've turned the tables on him. His fellow coauthors asked him to answer questions on the investment climate surrounding telemedicine as we near the end of the public health emergency.

We present this interview in a more traditional Q&A fashion to preserve Jared's responses in their entirety.

Q: *How have investors' attitudes toward healthcare tech changed from before COVID, during COVID, and as the COVID public health emergency (PHE) ends?*

A: Based on my experience, research, and many conversations with investment bankers, healthcare innovation has always been a large market. However, from 2019 to 2020, expansion-stage deals exploded. They doubled from $8.3 billion to $17.4 billion.[3] Prior to the PHE, investment in tech centered heavily on electronic medical record (EMR) systems, practice management software, marketing software, payer management, revenue cycle, and a few cases of telehealth (e.g., Teladoc, doctor on demand).

Yet as so often discussed throughout this book, the PHE brought telehealth into focus. One of the most notable investments was SoftBank's $300 million stake in Cerebral for a $4.8 billion valuation.[4] Meanwhile, massive investments in telehealth happened all across the board in 2020 and 2021 because of low interest rates (in the United States especially) and an immediate need for services. Most interestingly, investors were utterly comfortable investing in highly unprofitable companies that would eventually turn a profit to get in early on the telehealth "land grab."

As the PHE ends and interest rates increase, we are experiencing an *overindulgence* of telehealth investments. Valuations are leveling out and investors are seeking profitable companies with solid financial situations. This is a pendulum swing back to times before the PHE. The big difference is that many of these companies that raised large amounts during the PHE are now overvalued.

Many are predicting flat, down rounds or market consolidation just for companies to continue operating.[5] Indeed, we're already seeing many of these high-profile companies lay off a significant portion of their headcount to stabilize balance sheets, including Cerebral.[6]

Q: *Why is the end of the PHE so important to investors and how will it affect telehealth companies?*

A: The end of the PHE has many implications for healthcare companies, particularly on the telehealth side. Remote medicine as a concept has been around for decades, as we have covered in these pages. However, the 2008 Ryan Haight Act made it illegal to prescribe controlled substances solely via telehealth. Meanwhile the regulatory bodies of healthcare, like the DEA, CMS, and state medical boards, all focus on location-based management.

The PHE changed that. Prior to the PHE, practitioners needed individual medical licenses and DEA registrations in every state. These regulatory bodies loosened regulations, allowing for cross-border services to prescribe controlled substances or (generally) see patients out-of-state. This enabled doctors from California to support underserved populations in, say, Mississippi.

The end of the PHE removes many of the regulatory relaxations. Practitioners will suddenly be required to have a DEA in every state they operate. At the same time, each state will require an in-state medical license tied to a practice location, and often a secondary controlled substance registration. On top of that, the DEA will again require at least one in-person visit prior to prescribing controlled substances.

The big change is the *perception* of these laws. "Meet the patient where they are" is the motto of many telehealth practices these days.

Patients love it. If these regulatory bodies remove that ability, we will all suffer from a massive decrease in affordable care. For investors, this means their belief in telehealth could be undercut by requiring in-person models, as these will significantly increase real estate, personnel, and regulatory costs. It will transform the modality of telehealth from "completely virtual" to "hybrid." Of course, the market will have vast uncertainty until things normalize, which could take years.

Q: *How has valuation for telehealth companies been affected by the current financial situation?*

A: Healthcare is usually one of the more stable markets in the U.S. Everybody needs it, and large institutions own most of the sector. Telehealth is unique because a plethora of start-ups have disrupted the space, and large hospital systems have been financially challenged over the last few years.[7] Also, low interest rates have made the cost of capital relatively cheap, so investors could raise large rounds at low interest rates.

With an increase of interest rates, capital cost has gone up, thus funding for telehealth companies has become scarcer. Adding to the uncertainty at the end of the PHE and the regulatory "Wild West" companies enjoyed, valuations have decreased. They will continue to remain low until market clarity occurs. This *already* means layoffs and down rounds, but it could also include consolidation and the closure of companies, uncommon in healthcare.

Q: *What are current market drivers in healthcare tech?*

A: There are several in the healthcare tech marketplace. Growth is always critical for any company, but also profitability and sound balance sheets. At the same time, since U.S. healthcare is highly fragmented (particularly in telehealth) and there are large mergers, consolidation seems like it will increasingly be a driver, in 2024 and beyond.

The other drivers that I have heard regularly discussed are business aspects. If a company can add or bolster tech, that can be a win. If investors see a chance to accelerate growth, that's likely a driver. Likewise, if a company is trying to hedge against market volatility, that can also be a driver. However, each of these are more situationally dependent on the investor needs and the overall health tech sector.

Q: *How do companies stand out to investors in the current marketplace?*

A: Right now, profitable companies with strong balance sheets are obviously the most attractive. As well, companies with strong, long-term contracts with payers or government institutions (i.e., the Veterans Association) are considered more favorable.

Q: *What should investors expect in three to five years in healthcare tech?*

A: It's unlikely anyone really knows what will happen based on the marketplace's current turbidity. However, a few trends seem likely. Patients now expect telehealth as an alternative to in-person care. So telehealth is not going away (though it may look different).

Second, as remote monitoring tech improves, we will see a further integration between hardware and healthcare. Whether someone is tracking their sleep with the Oura Ring or monitoring their heart rate with the Apple Watch, remote monitoring will progress steadily. The question becomes: "What to do with all of that data?" For instance, what happens if you're receiving a live feed of a patient experiencing signs of pre-heart-attack conditions? Is it the provider's responsibility to proactively assess the risk and react?

Last, in-person healthcare will continue to exist in many situations. We all know you cannot repair a gunshot wound or have a baby remotely. That won't change anytime soon.

Q: *We keep hearing how the big tech companies (Meta, Google, Amazon, Apple, and Microsoft) are trying to break into healthcare, but it seems like a lot of their initiatives have failed to take off. Why do you think that is? Why is it so hard for companies to disrupt healthcare?*

A: Honestly, I don't think some of them are trying to "win" healthcare. Rather, they wish to take a slice relating to their core or near-adjacent business. Microsoft wants hospitals to run on Azure or maybe use D365 for fundraising. That's not going to disrupt healthcare, but they can make meaningful revenue from that space. Apple wants to sell more watches and phones. Health data is a way to do that (and probably the best use case for their watch). When it comes to Google, they have made a larger healthcare foray. Their strategy seems to be focused on piloting every large industry, but always returning to their core products: search, data, and cloud.

Amazon is the most interesting major player. They are trying to build their own health plan via buying a hybrid telehealth/primary care company (One Medical) and establishing a remote prescription-filling business. I wouldn't rule out Amazon on that front. They're currently piloting most of this vertical approach to their employees to reduce healthcare costs and, when ready, they will try to take on the general market.

But there are very large players to compete with, and healthcare, unlike Amazon's core business of "anything that fits in a box," is complex. For instance, what's the price of a brain surgery? Still, overall, some combination of Whole Foods, One Medical, and Amazon's ability to operationalize well can offer an opportunity for hybrid clinics in the future.

LOOKING AHEAD

Although telemedicine's immediate future is uncertain to investors, the core concept behind it has been a dramatic success. One reason QuickMD has succeeded so well so fast is by bringing lifesaving care to those who lost hope in our legacy healthcare system. It's our wish the coming years expand the horizons of what's possible, leading to better health outcomes via tech. In our next chapter, we look at doctors pioneering the art of wellness through telemedicine—instead of just treating patients when they are ill.

CHAPTER 11

Telehealth Isn't Just for Sick People—It's a Wellness Boon

Jeremy Martinez was only in his early thirties and already a rising star at one of the most powerful Silicon Valley start-ups. After six years of climbing the ranks, he was a power player in the org chart. He carried heavy responsibilities related to product innovation, hitting revenue goals, and leading multiple design teams. Every move Jeremy made affected the careers and financial security of more than 1,500 talented employee reports. This responsibility was both a privilege and a burden. The latter especially.

Being in charge of so many affected Jeremy's health. He started thinking about this subject more after recent corporate reorganization. His company's own "skunkworks"—industry speak for a team that works on secret projects most of their own peers don't even know exist—was reassigned to Jeremy's leadership. Practically, that meant he got to visit clandestine company labs, learning about cutting-edge projects. Many were considered to be "moonshot" grades. They featured groundbreaking ideas that could transform life for people the world over.

To say Jeremy was blown away by what he saw on a recent tour would be an understatement. Experts he affectionately calls "mad scientists" showed him a prototype of a wearable much like his own smartwatch. It tracks blood glucose levels without the need for finger pricks and testing strips, or direct blood contact of any sort. The wearable has an AI monitor to alert wearers when their blood sugar reaches a dangerous level. It can also automatically summon help if it hits a critical level.

As the mad scientists perfected their new product, they'd begun considering more blood chemistry analysis using the same device. Jeremy, for his part, could not help but think of his diabetic cousin and how this innovation could improve—if not save—her life. The mad scientists also showed Jeremy another wearable to measure the breathing of infants and the critically ill. Sound collected via a sensitive yet unobtrusive microphone array can not only gauge a patient's breathing function but also create a sonic map of the lungs so doctors can make more informed treatment decisions. Jeremy was stunned. "You mean to tell me the rest of this company has been killing itself dreaming up better headphones at the same time you guys were changing the world?"

One of the mad scientists, Dr. Nwadike, said, "Jeremy, don't take it so hard. The innovations your teams have developed *enable* these advances. And without millions of people buying the headphones and other devices you all design, none of the work you've just seen could be funded."

In the ensuing months, the more Jeremy learned about his employer's underground initiatives, the more determined he got to take care of his own health. He wanted to be sound enough to stick around until these inventions (and others still on the drawing board) came alive. Working for another decade in such a career might not seem like such a challenge for someone in their early 30s, but Silicon Valley is not a normal workplace.

Jeremy knew this well. He had seen what had happened to older people working both at his company and at others nearby. Burnout rates shot sky-high because of intense work schedules. More troublingly, he observed how the longer seasoned execs continued working, the more they felt they must work even *harder* to keep up with the limitless energy of fresh graduates. Jeremy was already feeling the pinch of this exhaustion after only six years. Watching so many others crash and burn, he knew he didn't want to end up like them.

Often, Jeremy's mind would drift to such cautionary tales. He observed many bright stars dimmed from overwork. Yes, they might have earned millions and millions of dollars, but they also paid a price for their wealth. All had health conditions. A few had even suffered from heart attacks or strokes at a young age. This disturbed Jeremy so much that he went to his dad to ask, "What good is it making $5 million a year if you can't even enjoy it?"

"That sounds like a curse, not a blessing."

Jeremy knew his dad was right. So he set out to assess his current health level with an eye on improving it. The last thing he wanted to do was end up a rich guy with a broken-down body (or mind!). As a relentlessly analytical business executive, Jeremy turned to the one tool he consistently used to determine the scope of any new project: a SWOT analysis. SWOT stands for strengths, weaknesses, opportunities, and threats. Assessing this way allowed Jeremy to place different factors into each category, prioritizing actions for any successful product launch.

In this case? The product launch is a lifetime of good health.

Right away, Jeremy listed several strengths. He had never had a major injury or illness. He also did not take prescriptions besides the Adderall. His physical activity level was good. He went to a gym three days a week and often found opportunities during his busy day to build movement into the course of his work—for example, using a standing desk and walking in a nearby park at lunch.

Our young executive then listed weaknesses. He knew his work-life balance was out of whack. Once upon a time, he worked crazy hours only during "crunch time" like before a product launch. However, crunch time had morphed into all the time as his career progressed. He also marked down drug usage. Jeremy relied on caffeine to start his day. He enjoyed moderate amounts of alcohol on social occasions, but he regularly used other substances, too. Like many a tech gladiator, he turned to Adderall to enhance his concentration and focus. He didn't know what the long-term effect of this may be but doubted it was healthy. Jeremy also wasn't sleeping enough, sometimes just four hours a night, resorting to sleeping pills to take the edge off his afternoon Adderall.

When it came to opportunities, Jeremy had to think hard. This part of his SWOT analysis concerned what he could do to improve his situation. After some contemplation, he came up with a plan: Find a physical trainer willing to accommodate his chaotic schedule. Jeremy also wanted to investigate meal prep services to eat better. His normal lunch was prepared by company chefs onsite, but he tended to skip breakfast or eat fast food on the way to work, and dinner could be all over the map.

Finally, he moved to threats. Possible dangers to Jeremy's health were clear. Work stress, burnout risk, and the gnawing fear that he couldn't keep up with the competition in a cutthroat industry all weighed on his mind. Yet he considered his single greatest threat to be lack of time. He was often double-booked in meetings and habitually overloaded with progress reports and other paperwork. How could he accomplish *anything* health related without adding more hours to his day? Hours he didn't have.

At first, Jeremy thought he was done with his analysis. Then, he picked his pen back up, reconsidering more opportunities. He had listed a variety of professionals like a personal trainer who could help him improve his physical fitness, but he had left another type of professional out—what about seeing a doctor?

Until now, our young executive never had much time for physicians. In his mind, that's who you see when you're sick, not when you're well. But recent events had made him realize this approach might be wrong. Beyond his special projects division explaining how wearables and continuous monitoring can catch problems before they escalate, Jeremy had also seen senior professionals keeping personal doctors on staff for checkups and lifestyle direction, though many were young and healthy.

Jeremy added seeing a doctor to his list of opportunities, but he still considered it to be a challenge. It's not like he was high enough up the food chain to afford a personal doctor, like Mark Zuckerberg and other tech titans. He also couldn't afford to lose half a workday traveling to an MD's office. Deciding to tackle this issue before taking on other things he listed, Jeremy did what so many an executive does whenever they feel stuck—he turned to his resourceful executive assistant, Sarah.

After explaining his dilemma, he asked for the impossible: locate a nearby doctor to see him quickly and help him plan for a healthier life. Sarah got to work. The next morning, she greeted Jeremy with a bright smile. "I've found the perfect doctor. His name is Dr. Sam Lavis, and he practices functional medicine. He uses nutrition and other treatments to maintain total body health. *Proactively*."

Jeremy was thrilled. "Great. I assume you scheduled an appointment a few weeks out so I can take half a day off."

Sarah's smile grew even brighter. "Oh, you're seeing him today."

"Huh?" Jeremy looked at her like she'd just grown another head. "How'd you swing that? Anyway, I've got a product review at 10:00, an executive presentation at 3:00, and a factory visit at 6:00. I can't travel to a doctor—even one 20 minutes away."

Sarah's smile never faded. "You don't have to *travel* to see Dr. Lavis. He uses telemedicine. I scheduled an appointment with him during your 30 minutes of downtime after product review. You can take the appointment from your office. No travel needed."

Jeremy wasn't sold on the idea, but he trusted Sarah. She'd never steered him wrong. Still, as he went about his morning routine, he couldn't help but wonder just how useful this would prove to be.

Before long, it was time to meet Dr. Lavis.

When Jeremy got on the app Sarah downloaded, he noticed one important factor. He felt more comfortable on his office couch than in any typical doctor's office. He also liked how promptly the connection occurred. Within seconds of logging in, Dr. Lavis greeted him. "Jeremy, I understand you're concerned about preserving your health. I keep patients healthy by being mindful of what every system in the body does. Let's work together to make that happen for you."

Instantly, Jeremy knew Sarah had knocked it out of the park.

During that first appointment, Jeremy also noted how Dr. Lavis didn't rush him along like so many caregivers he'd seen before. Instead, he spent time getting to know his new patient. They even discussed everything Jeremy recorded in his SWOT analysis, from exercise levels to sleep to diet to drug use. At length they also went over Jeremy's family history of illness, including relatives who suffered from heart disease. Like with any productive meeting in Jeremy's career, he came away with some homework assignments.

First, Jeremy was to stop by a lab minutes from his office to have blood drawn for Dr. Lavis's advanced testing. Jeremy was comfortable with this, especially as it involved no waiting. Knowing Jeremy was so time sensitive, Dr. Lavis first explained, "You won't be held up by a lack of resources. You'll be in the door, get blood drawn, and be back on your way." Additionally, the doctor asked Jeremy to pick up an Oura Ring. "It'll help us track your sleeping."

Most importantly, Jeremy felt good about the plan to manage his health Dr. Lavis had laid out. Following this introductory period, Jeremy was to see his new doctor via telemedicine every two weeks. After the blood test data came back and the sleep tracker provided significant, actionable data, Dr. Lavis would create a tailored health plan for Jeremy, a personalized road map to health that they would continuously assess and tweak.

Soon, Jeremy felt more in control of his health than ever before. For its part, the sleep tracker identified dramatic shortfalls in restful sleep that Jeremy had neglected for years. Soon after, he could predict what days he could expect to have more energy than usual. He started prioritizing getting more rest. Moreover, the advanced bloodwork Dr. Lavis ordered showed inflammatory blood markers, leading to a robust nutrition plan for increasing protein while minimizing foods contributing to problems.

Several months into his new health journey, Jeremy felt better than he could recall feeling. He also got more done in a day than he had in years. His superiors noticed he was achieving new productivity levels—all without depending on drugs to stay sharp. Importantly, Jeremy's frequent meetings with Dr. Lavis did not interfere with his work schedule or cause him stress from having to take time off to travel to a doctor's office. Put simply, telemedicine revitalized his well-being, offering him a renewed sense of vitality and purpose.

CONCIERGE MEDICINE IN THE TELEHEALTH AGE

The story you've just read is based on a real patient; only personal details have been changed to protect privacy. One aspect that wasn't changed is the name of the physician, Dr. Sam Lavis. He's a real doctor remotely assisting patients across the nation. Before the COVID-19 pandemic made telehealth a viable care option, Dr. Lavis contemplated how to positively disrupt the legacy care model. He developed a passion for peak performance in high school, leading to an interest in functional medicine.

The Institute for Functional Medicine (IFM) defines functional medicine as "a systems biology–based approach that focuses on identifying and addressing the root cause of disease. Each symptom or differential diagnosis may be one of many contributing to an individual's illness."[1] Under this view of health, a mental issue like depression may be traced back to physiological causes, such as vitamin D deficiency. Meanwhile, one such cause can result in many deleterious health outcomes, such as inflammation contributing to arthritis and even heart disease.

Board certified in family medicine, Dr. Lavis attended Pacific Northwest University for medical school, serving a rotation in the prestigious Cleveland Clinic's Functional Medicine Program.[2] This training prepared him to be an excellent functional medicine doctor, but telemedicine is what empowered Dr. Lavis to achieve the type of care he envisioned back in high school. The authors sat down with Dr. Lavis to discuss how practicing at the edge of this emerging field is helping patients wake up to the value of concierge healthcare.

Maintaining Contact Is Key

We began by exploring why Dr. Lavis feels it matters to be in regular contact with patients. "In medical school and residency, I did rotations with functional doctors. They would often charge patients significant amounts for an in-depth initial consultation, then meet with them one more time after six months. I saw patients who stagnated under this model, and it bothered me. It made me want to practice differently: to be more involved in their health *every* step of the way. Accountability and other positive things tend to come from consistent follow-up, especially with patients and caregivers working in tandem. For most of my patients, biweekly check-ins offer the perfect mechanism to get this right."

Dr. Lavis elaborates on why these follow-ups are so critical. "No one is going to improve their health based on one visit and a six-month check-in. Realistically, we know it takes four to six months to begin to see improvement in health due to nutrition changes and other lifestyle shifts, but that means four to six months of *following the program*. The only thing that made sense was to design one whereby a patient can follow up with me as often as needed, and I can follow up with them too."

Similar to the tale of Jeremy, functional medicine isn't only about getting over illnesses. Dr. Lavis explains, "With every patient, one of the first things we do is advanced lab testing, akin to a colonoscopy for the blood. In this assessment, we're looking for signs like abnormal nutrition markers, inflammatory indicators, and cardiac risks that probably wouldn't show up on a standard blood test. This helps us avoid chronic illnesses that might appear 10 to 15 years down the road. That's especially crucial for younger patients who want to enjoy their later years."

Based on the findings of such testing, Dr. Lavis creates a plan tailored to the patient and their goals. Regular follow-ups matter to this process, especially as a plan may need to be modified based on patient performance. Dr. Lavis explains, "We often start by improving diet instead of jumping right into medicine. Depending on how a patient is doing after month one or two, we can introduce supplements and medication. The same thing goes for men with low testosterone levels. We don't necessarily try to correct the issue right away, because it may correct itself as diet shifts. If the patient is struggling six weeks into the program, we can, of course, course correct."

Dr. Lavis sees value in telemedicine for facilitating the type of care he practices characterized by frequent check-ins. He expands on such value, saying, "I am talking to the typical functional medicine patient every two weeks. It would be crazy to expect them to come to an office that often, though. Some have the luxury of time to pull this schedule off, but we've found it simply isn't needed. Instead, we can have just as good of a conversation—if not better—with the patient sitting in a comfortable environment they know and connecting to me via an app. In fact, the patient's comfort level makes a typical telehealth appointment more productive than an in-person visit, in my opinion."

He continues, "Like Jeremy, some of my patients are executives at major tech and industrial companies. They don't have the bandwidth to drop everything and see a doctor regularly. But they do have time to hop on a telemedicine app and talk to me about their successes and challenges with the program. The consistency and accountability of these regular telehealth appointments drive positive patient outcomes. With businesspeople in general, they do well with virtual meetings because they do them so often. I use the share screen function to show them lab reports, and they're in their element."[3]

Telemedicine Jump-Started His Practice

At age 31, Dr. Lavis had another practical reason for turning to telemedicine beyond its ability to empower frequent follow-ups. The modality also facilitated building his burgeoning practice. "Realistically, not every patient is interested in functional medicine. There are plenty of people who just want to get a prescription and feel better. I knew I would be much more effective in building my own career if I could reach patients interested in proactively managing their health in a far wider area than just my small town in Washington state. Telemedicine is what enabled this. Only one-third of my practice is local. The other two-thirds are spread out across the state and throughout the U.S. Right now, 75% of my appointments occur via telemedicine. I don't see that dropping in the future."

Dr. Lavis also believes his young age gave him a strong professional foundation. "Part of my residency focused on telemedicine due to COVID-19. So, in a sense, my training was in remote care while older doctors trained in the legacy way. Also, many doctors worry about hitting criteria for insurance billing that can be tough to accommodate through telehealth, but my practice is largely based on a *subscription model*, so I'm not worried about jumping through insurance hoops—just on improving my patients' lives."

Unlike more traditional caregivers, Dr. Lavis's practice bills directly to patients. He offers varying price points to fit different budgets, ranging from a basic service, including access to him to ask medical questions, all the way to a much more extensive plan in which Dr. Lavis designs specific meals and exercise regimens. He also experiments with new techniques, such as bringing 10 to 12 people together via Zoom to discuss their struggles and challenges in a group setting, much like a remote mastermind. "Patients can find benefits just from hearing someone else's story," he explains.

Telemedicine's (Small) Downside and (Big) Upside

We next asked Dr. Lavis to describe what he sees as the largest drawback to practicing in his telemedicine style. It's a matter of work-life balance. "My patients have access to my phone, Zoom, and other contact methods, so boundaries can get blurred. As functional medicine patients start to excel with their plan, they often want to get in touch with me as their doctor instead of dreading visits. This is a challenge right now."

He deals with this by setting patient expectations. Dr. Lavis must explain to patients they won't get an immediate answer from him in the evenings, or in early mornings for those on the East Coast. "It's a matter of setting limits. Most people are reasonable about it because they know I'm their doctor, not some giant corporation. Still, no matter what I do, there will be the occasional calls on a Saturday, but those are typically legitimate situations where I don't mind being contacted."

This downside pales in comparison to the upsides of telehealth in his opinion. "What I enjoy most about this model is I can provide an excellent standard of care to more patients in a way that's easier to accommodate. Especially those professionals like Jeremy who are on the go. And technology is improving all the time. I don't think a week goes by without hearing something exciting about what we can do next with health."

On the day of our interview, Dr. Lavis explained he was about to meet with a rep of a company offering remote assessment for blood pressure that also offers consumer-friendly EKG systems and continuous glucose monitoring (CGM) devices.[4] The service allows patients to monitor their body at home with the data going directly to Dr. Lavis. He explains what impact such technological advances have on him as a practicing physician. "It's actually fun, learning how to make this process more efficient, more effective, and less of a burden on the patient. These types of advancements make it ever easier for patients to contribute to their own health in new, empowering ways."

As the father of a young child, Dr. Lavis also sees advantages for parents to improve their professional work-life balance, thanks to telemedicine. "I'm busy building my practice right now, but in the near future I plan to enjoy one day a week where I don't have appointments. I will be available if patients need me, but that day will offer extra time to spend with my family. I could never do that if I was purely a bricks-and-mortar-type doctor."

QuickMD frequently hears from our female physicians that schedule flexibility and the ability to balance the needs of their kids with work have been a key driver in their professional success since joining us. As the parent of a young child, Dr. Lavis shares a similar experience. In fact, the week before our interview he had the type of day that telemedicine now helps doctors manage.

"The sitter who watches my son on Wednesdays couldn't take him. I was supposed to have a patient coming into the office, but I asked them to meet via Zoom, which they were happy to do. I could work right from home while my son did his own thing in the same room. In fact, a few patients asked me to bring him on camera to say hello. It wasn't an ideal situation because I had to keep an eye on him, but I completed my work *and* addressed my patients' needs instead of canceling on them. I can only imagine this type of flexibility is even more important for physicians who are also moms."

The Future of Telemedicine

Dr. Lavis sees bright days ahead. "Functional medicine in particular, and many other care areas in general, will turn heavily toward this model going forward. There will always be patients, especially the elderly, who prefer in-person visits, but most people like telehealth because it's easier. In my practice, I see a strong desire for concierge services. High-achieving people want this flexibility. *They need it*. They are high achieving for a reason—they are extremely busy."

Dr. Lavis is also excited for the future of wearables and continuous monitoring. "We're getting to the point where my patients can have devices like the Oura Ring, a scale, a CGM, and other devices feeding data directly to me. They don't need to go to an office or anywhere else for me to gather these vital signs. Instead, I get the data as needed, and

I can review it when necessary. I'm not to the point where I'm reaching out to clients proactively based on readings I'm seeing, but I know it's approaching. From a health perspective, it's great to imagine a patient learning about a blood pressure problem fast, instead of waiting a full year between checkups to know something's up. Also, these readings will be far more accurate when taken during sleep rather than in the office, like the data coming off the Oura Ring."[5]

Clearly, Dr. Sam Lavis is blazing a new trail in telemedicine. He's using this new model to break down needless barriers to patient success, particularly in the world of functional medicine. His work is also expanding care availability by helping (many overscheduled) patients fit healthcare into their busy lives. But far beyond his particular field, telemedicine is also having a similarly positive effect in making doctors' visits more accessible to underserved populations. We shall cover this development now.

TELEHEALTH MAKES HEALTHCARE MORE EQUITABLE

It should surprise no one that the COVID-19 pandemic drove patient willingness to see a doctor via telemedicine higher. In a November 2022 article, *U.S. News and World Report* explained just how far we've swung toward telehealth.[6] According to data gathered by the RAND American Life Panel and first published in the journal *Health Affairs*, desire to use a video-based telehealth service soared from 51 percent of Americans in 2019 to 62 percent in 2021. But the more startling data comes from historically underserved populations, and the picture painted is a huge win for healthcare equity.[7]

According to the RAND data, inclinations to use telemedicine among Black adults rose from 42 percent in 2019 to 67 percent in 2021.[8] In other words, Black Americans who were once far less likely to adopt remote care are now *more willing* than the general population to turn to telemedicine. This development promises to close the care gap that still exists in minority communities.[9]

Already, the healthcare industry understands the role telemedicine can play in improving health equity. Sheri Dodd, vice president and general manager of Medtronic Care Management Systems, explains in a recent interview that "one of the outcomes of COVID-19 was a greater awareness that we are overly reliant on a very old school way of delivering care. That wasn't viable during COVID-19 and it's not a sustainable, equitable delivery model."[10]

Dodd elaborated on the medical device giant's future plans, saying that it would pursue strategic and creative partnerships with telecommunications platforms to "unlock the full power of digital technologies to help serve patients," regardless of their location and health needs.[11]

A similar parity exists among Americans who are not highly educated. In 2019, 30 percent of adults without a high school education were willing to consider telehealth. In 2021, that figure leapt to 56 percent.[12] In many cases, less educated people are also likely to be economically underprivileged, making affordable treatment that doesn't involve hiring a babysitter or taking time off work a key component to improving one's health.

To be sure, these patients face a different problem than our tech executive who enjoyed success with Dr. Lavis because he didn't have to divert his career to be healthy—these are people who desperately need an improved system to give them better options for seeking basic care.

TELEHEALTH MEANS MORE REGULAR CARE FOR CHRONIC CONDITIONS

A recent white paper by the Agency for Healthcare Research and Quality (AHRQ) presents clear findings of the positive impacts on healthcare that telemedicine brings to the table. It states, "There is a large volume of research reporting that clinical outcomes with telehealth are as good as or better than usual care and that telehealth improves intermediate outcomes and satisfaction." It also lays out three key areas in which telemedicine is specifically useful:

- Remote, home monitoring for patients with chronic conditions, such as chronic obstructive pulmonary disease and congestive heart failure
- Communicating and counseling patients with chronic conditions
- Providing psychotherapy as part of behavioral health[13]

Already, we have seen these applications echoed throughout this book. Here are prime examples:

- TeleMAT for opioid addiction
- Home monitoring for an elderly dementia patient
- Psychiatrists using telehealth for High Fidelity Wraparound care to at-risk teens

The AHRQ also makes another important point about telemedicine's upsides—its quickness cannot be matched. "Impact occurs when speed matters."[14] Included in the discussion are life-threatening conditions like a heart attack in which ECG data can be sent ahead to the hospital. But this same concept applies to the care QuickMD supplies daily to patients. To someone suffering from opioid addiction, having to wait two weeks for a MAT appointment or being forced to travel hours to seek care can be a life-or-death matter. The fact that patients can now seek TeleMAT treatment from the comfort of their own homes again reduces needless barriers and saves lives.

This report came out in 2020 just as we were launching QuickMD. We believe if the agency was to study telemedicine just three years after its initial assessment, it would find an even more positive environment. Whether a patient is fighting addiction, requires basic medical care, or seeks the concierge care Dr. Sam Lavis provides, the clear answer is telemedicine. Remote care offers accurate, ongoing, easily accessible care for patients from all walks of life. It is particularly beneficial for those who wish to perform at their peak and optimize their lifestyle while avoiding long doctor's office wait times and infrequent check-ups. A net positive for all stakeholders indeed. As more doctors from more specialties come to embrace telemedicine and more tech companies introduce revolutionary medical devices, our view of the future of telemedicine is simple—*the sky's the limit.*

In our final chapter, we explore how even the sky may *not* be the limit for telemedicine's future. We explore what remote telemedicine can offer both patients and doctors alike when we someday live and work off-world.

CHAPTER 12

Telemedicine . . . in Space

A Dream Chaser space plane named *Tenacity* carries Caroline Ko into the relative calm of low-Earth orbit (LEO). A materials researcher specialist, Caroline just experienced a bumpy ride through our atmosphere at the top of a massive launch vehicle. While doing so, she reflected on how her own career has been bumpier than most might suspect.

Distinguishing herself in high school, she had her heart set on MIT. Unfortunately, the prestigious university didn't feel her achievements were enough to earn a scholarship. Instead of quitting, Caroline worked nights and weekends in her parents' Korean restaurant. She also redoubled her classroom efforts. She kept it up, working her fingers to the bone throughout her first year of college. All that changed once MIT learned they did, in fact, have something special on their hands.

You see, Caroline proved herself to be a gifted scientist *and* an engineer capable of developing innovative approaches to difficult problems in the world of cutting-edge materials. As PhD candidates and researchers puzzled over head-scratching conundrums, like how to apply a blend of exotic metals to reduce electrical fire dangers in airplanes, Caroline revealed herself more than capable of visualizing the solution in her head. Her academic career took off like a proverbial rocket, one that would later launch her into actual space.

Who would have thought this success would introduce its own set of problems? At 19, Caroline felt the weight of the world on her shoulders. Professors pressured her to help their research projects succeed. Meanwhile, older students resented the newcomer overshadowing their work. Caroline wasn't out to outshine anybody—she maintained a humble attitude and supported everyone she could. Even so, hostility from others in her department nearly made her quit.

But a visit with her grandmother after sophomore year convinced Caroline to stick with it. During summer vacation with extended family, Caroline opened up to her grandmother about her troubles. The latter listened with sympathy before sharing wisdom Caroline would recall for the rest of her life. "Those people in your lab are worried because they think you are a backstabber in a long line of academic backstabbers. But they don't know your heart. You owe it to yourself, your family, and to God to use your gifts to your fullest extent. If they treat you bad, meet them with a smile. No one can resist that beautiful smile of yours."

Bolstered by the pep talk, Caroline approached her junior and senior years with new resolve. She found a mentor in renowned materials scientist and professor Reginald Washington. Together, they formed a close working relationship. Often, he invited her into his home, where Caroline would join Reggie (as his students knew him), his wife, and their children Aaliyah and Lemarcus for dinner.

As Caroline approached graduation, she expected to continue her studies, first earning a master's degree and then a PhD. That plan changed one fortuitous day when she was in the lab setting up an experiment on a metallic crystalline material known as TN-1428. The exotic substance would later gain a flashy trade name at the commercialization stage. For now? Few people outside of the lab team knew it existed.

That morning Reggie burst in, bubbling with enthusiasm. "You won't believe the news I just got."

Without looking up, Caroline calmly responded, "Careful, Reggie. If you make me jump, this whole lab could go up in flames."

Her mentor wasn't fazed. "We've got big things cooking. I just met with the university bigwigs; they're forming a joint venture with a Silicon Valley company to explore TN-1428. They want to know how far we can take this stuff in microgravity." He added theatrical emphasis to the last word.

"Microgravity?" She finally looked up. "Where on earth can they set up a lab without gravity?"

"That's just it. *In space*, Caroline. They can place it outside our atmosphere. They want me to go to orbit and develop the tech to see if it can improve battery life. I told them I'd go, but only if I can bring my right-hand woman. What do you say?"

Caroline sat in stunned silence. *Me? Go to space? I'm no astronaut.*

Yet as fast as these thoughts appeared, she dismissed them. Reggie had been the key to her academic career. She wasn't about to miss this chance, not after he was so excited he was practically bouncing off the walls. She also had the confidence to believe her grandmother was right. She owed it to herself to seize this chance. "If we can safely live and work in space, I'm in."

Six months of busy preparation followed that split-second decision. Caroline and her mentor went through exercises and simulations in an earthbound copy of the Large Integrated Flexible Environment (LIFE) Habitat.[1] (This would be their home away from home for their four months in orbit.) She soon got used to the size of their diminutive living quarters and work environment while practicing safety procedures and picking up basics, like how to use the bathroom and brush your teeth in microgravity. She also learned the different roles aboard a space station. (Specialist astronauts like her who come from the private sector and perform R&D work in space differ from professional astronauts tasked with keeping everything running.)

The training also included a battery of medical tests to ensure a safe trip. At one point she met the telemedicine doctors she would regularly check in with from space. (Astronauts knowledgeable about first aid would be onboard, but no doctor.) This meant in the event of illness or other medical situation, telemedicine would provide initial care. Caroline was already comfortable with remote medicine from having grown up with it. She formed a bond with one team member in particular, Dr. Iris Kim. She felt a quick kinship with the young Korean doctor, even as she hoped not to need her services while in orbit.

The night before takeoff, Reggie found Caroline hunched over her laptop. "You're not *still* working? You must rest."

She looked up. "No, not working. I promised to help my cousin apply for financial aid to go to Caltech. I thought it better to do it before we left."

Reggie grinned at her. "Well, the Wi-Fi is pretty good up there, but I don't blame you for helping your family. Telling them, 'Sorry, I'm blasting off in a rocket tomorrow' does seem like a reasonable excuse, though. Anyhow, I'm gonna get some sleep before countdown."

Reggie and Caroline's flight went off without a hitch.

The Dream Chaser space plane launched from Earth Base One, Sierra Space's launch facility in Cape Canaveral, Florida. Before they knew it, the space station that would become their home swam into view. Officially named Orbital Base 13, or OB-13, it went by the moniker "the bakery" because it was the thirteenth Sierra Space orbital station. It consisted of five connected LIFE Habitats to create a sprawling facility dotted with solar panels and other modules for life support, facilitating R&D and other production activities.

The Dream Chaser docked gently with OB-13.

Caroline and Reggie checked out the station, identical to the simulator they had practiced in for months. Chief astronaut Jasmine Hawkins took them on a tour. As they clumsily floated along, she promised it would get easier after a few days. They stopped at the lab. It had been set up to Reggie's specifications, including a small saw to cut material samples into the correct shapes. Plastic surrounded the hook to prevent pieces of their experimental metals from contaminating systems and causing chaos with so much delicate electronics.

All and all, everything seemed to be in order.

Satisfied, the new arrivals went about the challenging task of unpacking in microgravity before dining with their new roommates. This station housed 30 astronauts in total, with most being specialists from academia and the private sector, like Caroline. Excited and nervous, she did her best to sleep later that first night, especially as she knew she had to make each day count.

Happily, Caroline and Reggie made amazing progress with TN-1428 the first week. They were both awed by the ease in which the material formed crystalline shapes impossible to construct on Earth. Caroline even grew used to hearing the saw's high-pitched whine as Reggie crafted pieces into shapes. They were thrilled because already at this early stage, it was obvious the material possessed the potential to disrupt industries, enabling a quantum leap forward in battery storage—among other industrial applications.

But not everything was perfect.

Caroline noticed Reggie didn't look well rested. He showed up in the mornings with bags under his eyes. He constantly had a coffee by his side in a squeeze pouch, quipping how his office mug wouldn't work too well in space. When she finally asked if he was having trouble sleeping, he admitted to some difficulty but said it was getting better. This wasn't true. Reggie was hardly sleeping at all, a common problem in LEO.

Neither knew this would soon lead to a full-blown crisis.

The next day, Reggie looked worse than ever as they floated into the lab. Busy with tests, Caroline was too distracted to notice. She didn't even look up when the whine of the saw started. Only Reggie's startled scream broke her concentration. With horror, she saw floating blood globules fill the lab. Reggie had badly cut himself and lost consciousness.

A warning klaxon sounded. The hatch sealed shut to prevent blood from contaminating the station. Only later would Caroline learn Reggie, who hadn't slept in practically a week, had finally fallen asleep. This caused him to slip forward and his arm to enter the saw's path.

Commander Hawkins appeared on Caroline's tablet in seconds. "You hurt too?"

Too shocked to be upset, Caroline replied, "N-No, just Reggie."

"Okay. Stand by for the doctor, I'm bringing her online now."

Caroline's friend Dr. Iris Kim appeared onscreen; her concern was apparent. "What happened?"

Caroline felt rising panic but managed to relate all she knew.

"Reggie will be okay, but he needs your help," said Dr. Kim calmly. "The lab is locked down until you can bring his bleeding under control. Do you know where he's hurt? If you don't see the wound, search for it now."

The doctor's reassuring tone spurred Caroline to action. Noticing Reggie's left arm coated in blood, she quickly found the wound. An ugly gash streaked all the way down to the bone.

"Found it. It's his forearm." She angled the tablet so Dr. Kim could see.

"Great job. Now, we must stop the bleeding."

"Should I tie a tourniquet?"

"That's our last resort. It will be hours before we can fit you into a spacesuit, undock, deorbit, and get you to a hospital. Leaving a tourniquet on so long would likely result in amputation. Instead, we must apply continuous direct pressure. Any ideas of what you can use nearby?"

Just as it had many times in labs on Earth, the solution to her dilemma appeared in Caroline's mind. "I've got an idea!"

She could use their latest batch of TN-1428.

Caroline got to work after first cleaning the wound with sterile fluid from the med kit. After just five minutes, she had created what looked like a thin bracelet. She got a perfect fit on her first try. The homemade medical device tightly covered the bleeding, instantly thwarting flow.

Next, Dr. Kim led Caroline through checks of Reggie's vital signs. It seemed like he was stable. With the bleeding stopped, the red alert was canceled and the door unlocked. Hawkins and others rushed in to render extra aid. They took Reggie to his quarters, where he awoke in major pain. Under Dr. Kim's direction, the crew gave him medication to stop the agony, saline via a special IV system, and antibiotics to prevent infection. Now, he just needed to wait until the emergency Dream Chaser flight home was available.

Caroline visited Reggie the next day.

"I finally got a good night's sleep," he confessed. Then he gestured to his arm where Caroline had stopped the bleeding using her experimental material. "This is amazing. I've been talking about it with Dr. Kim. The material stayed sterile, resistant to bacteria and seemingly everything else. Dr. Kim even thinks it encouraged faster clotting. You accidentally created the perfect bandage."

Forever humble, Caroline took the praise in stride. "What happens now?"

"I'm headed home. You'll stay on to continue our work until a replacement arrives. In the meantime? Tell your cousin to cancel his student loan request. You and Dr. Kim will have a share of the patent for this material. I don't think money will *ever* be a problem for you or your family again."

Stunned, Caroline could hardly process what her quick thinking meant for her future. Ever the practical scientist, she put the patent matter aside. She wished her mentor a speedy recovery and then headed out the hatch. She had a lab to clean and a full day's work to catch up on. Just as soon as she returned to Earth, she would meet Dr. Iris Kim in person. After working through an emergency together to such success, they owed each other at least that much.

TELEMEDICINE AND SPACE: A MATCH MADE IN THE HEAVENS?

Caroline's story is not exactly science fiction.

Sierra Space is a real company. The Dream Chaser space plane is on the verge of starting flights to low-Earth orbit. And we are only a few years away from private sector and academic researchers becoming specialist astronauts. These individuals will live and work in orbit aboard space stations constructed out of LIFE Habitats.[2] The company's ambitious plans to enable nonprofessionals to live and work in space has the potential to catapult innovation to incredible new heights in many areas, including energy, computing, manufacturing, and as we saw in Caroline's tale, medical tech.

Telemedicine will also be a major component to facilitating experts living and working off-world. Sans a full-time doctor aboard a space station—which is unlikely because of the low number of people aboard each station—a team of remote-based physicians on Earth will be needed. Even when things are running smoothly. In the case of an emergency like that suffered by Reggie in the lab, telemedicine will mean the difference between life and death.

To gain true insight into how telemedicine will affect private sector space exploration in this, our final chapter, we turned to an expert in this area. Dr. Thomas H. Marshburn has intimate knowledge and deep experience on both sides of this discussion. A medical doctor, at one point he served as the medical operations lead for the International Space Station

(ISS). At the same time, he is an astronaut with extensive space experience, including stints aboard the ISS. As part of SpaceX Crew-3, Marshburn spent 177 days in orbit aboard the ISS.[3] He also holds the record for oldest person to perform a spacewalk at 61.[4]

In 2022, Dr. Marshburn joined Sierra Space as chief medical officer (CMO) for the company's Human Spaceflight Center and Astronaut Training Academy.[5] His job is to train future astronauts while developing those policies and procedures to keep them safe and healthy in LEO. Consequently, there is perhaps no one more qualified to discuss the role telemedicine will play in humanity's off-planet future. The coauthors greatly enjoyed the opportunity to pick his brain about telehealth's final frontier.

WHAT REMOTE CARE WILL MEAN FOR SPACE

Sierra Space envisions a radical near future in which professionals such as scientists, engineers, and technicians live and work in the heavens. They dub this the Orbital Age, as it represents as large a leap forward as the Industrial or Computer Age. Since Dr. Marshburn has been a NASA flight surgeon and now serves as director of Sierra Space's program to prepare both professional astronauts and private-sector specialists, we began by asking him to explain telemedicine's importance in helping the Orbital Age come online.

"Everyone involved, from top to bottom, believes telehealth is essential to achieving humanity's goals in space," he explains. "Simply put, we won't be able to fly medical experts up to LEO whenever they are needed. It's just not practical or feasible. One of the main reasons telehealth is critical to the space economy is that flying to space is so disruptive to any doctor's career. Medical experts are authorities *because* they practice medicine daily. But if you're continually flying to space, you must become a jack of all trades. You'll have to become a crew member and do other things, like learn to fly the ship. As a doctor, I was also the pilot of NASA SpaceX Crew-3. I needed to wear many hats at the same time. We are embarking on a different era."

Next, Dr. Marshburn describes how training can affect a doctor's career. "Preparation for spaceflight is intense. A doctor can't see patients and practice medicine to the same degree when training for space travel. In fact, a doctor who's undergone spaceflight training will be out of practice within a year or so. In the future, when humans take long spaceflights, their skills may be out of date by two years or more before they're ever needed. These factors discourage doctors from spaceflight, and inevitably, in the future when we *do* have more doctors off-world, they will need to be in close contact with specialists on the ground."

We next asked Dr. Marshburn to explain the balance between what astronauts should be trained to help with medically, versus turning to remote support. According to him, astronauts must be ready to help with immediate first aid. In our fictional story, both Caroline and Reggie were locked in a lab by a safety system after a serious accident. They required immediate help from an Earth-based doctor, but what about the case of a crew member feeling ill?

Dr. Marshburn explains, "Astronauts are screened for preflight, so we're confident they're healthy. But nothing's foolproof. They can get appendicitis even if they are cleared for takeoff. All sorts of things can happen. Astronauts must therefore be trained to react immediately. If someone is choking in space, you don't have the time to get online. You must be able to perform the Heimlich maneuver—which presents its own set of challenges in microgravity."

"So we train for contingencies," he continues. "We cover topics like what to do if someone is choking, how to start CPR, where are the first aid kits and what is in them. In many cases we foster medical skills, like starting an IV. This is a medical procedure, but it's really a manual skill, so we practice it until astronauts are proficient. Ultimately, our goal is to continue the mission safely with our entire crew as healthy as possible. The worst thing that can happen is endangering lives and a multibillion-dollar mission because we lack certain basic skills telehealth can't help with in the heat of the moment."[6]

HOW TELEHEALTH RESPONDS TO SICKNESS AND ACCIDENTS IN SPACE

Next, we asked Dr. Marshburn to walk us through a potential scenario based on his experience as both a doctor and an astronaut. He laid out one his team has often used to refine their telemedicine approach. "What I think about a lot is the same challenge that confounds physicians in ERs daily: abdominal pain. This malady can run the whole spectrum, from simply needing to go to the bathroom to being a full-on emergency. There is never a clear answer. Always, some risk is associated with the decision we must make. So we've examined how this could occur on a Sierra Space mission in LEO."

He then laid out the scenario. "A crew member comes to the captain complaining of abdominal pain. There is no medical lab on the space station, but when he reviews the medical literature, the captain finds that lab values don't really help diagnose abdominal pain to any great degree anyway. He turns to a physical exam guided by a telemedicine doctor. Using the video link, a doctor can instruct the captain on how to perform the exam. At the same time, the Earth-based doctor can watch for subtle patient reactions. For example, if we're dealing with an abdominal abscess, the patient's abdomen will suddenly become rigid if the patient is bumped. (The captain or crewmember who is performing the exam might not understand the patient's reactions, but the doctor on the ground can derive tremendous insight from their video-based observations.)

"Based on this physical examination, if we're worried by what we're seeing, we will move on to an ultrasound machine," Dr. Marshburn continues. "This can feed data directly back to the people on the ground. If this ultrasound performed by the captain and/or crew—and guided by a doctor—confirms an abdominal abscess, we would likely start treatment with antibiotics using prior training on IV insertion. Last, if the situation requires it, we can perform minimally invasive procedures in space. Needle aspiration performed by crew could drain the abscess, relieving pressure. As you can imagine, the connection to a telehealth doctor would be crucial here."

As for the actual procedure, the telehealth physician monitoring the video and via the ultrasound would guide the captain and/or crewmember performing the needle biopsy. Doctors acting as telemedicine support for space crews would undergo specific training. In emergency situations, they will get the best results by understanding astronauts and how they relate to each other. Even down to their unique lexicon.

"I envision this surgery performed by an astronaut who would be guided by a telehealth physician using the same communication style. 'Pitch the needle up and rotate left' might not mean much to regular people, but to a pilot used to docking with a space station, they would know what must happen with that needle. In this scenario, the patient could be stabilized until a relief mission could be summoned. Now, in the case of a longer flight to Mars, other technologies would be needed—like more robust medical supplies, possibly an AI to monitor vitals and direct care when traveling so far from Earth."

Of course, as more people live and work in space, accidents will occur, similar to our speculative story. We asked Dr. Marshburn to explain how telehealth can aid in such situations. "When these happen, and I've personally dealt with lacerations in space, the first step is always to stop the bleeding. We needn't have complicated procedures that must be read in a crisis. Instead, we train astronauts to do what is most pragmatic. If the connection is made to a telehealth doctor immediately, they can help in this initial pressing capacity. Only afterward will they move to assessing the wound's severity."

He explains, "Just as on Earth, different types of wounds can result in different levels of concern. I've worked in ERs where car crash victims with scalp wounds think they will die due to the amount of blood from head wounds. Actually, they are quite okay. On the other hand, a thigh wound involving major blood vessels without obvious external bleeding is more dangerous. Whatever the specific case, the telehealth doctor can discern the appropriate way to deal with the wound. This may involve staples, sutures, or Dermabond, a type of wound adhesive. The crew can then wrap up the injury and in most cases, stabilize the patient."

PROTECTING ASTRONAUTS' MENTAL HEALTH

As outlined in this book, remote care is making major strides in this field. Astronauts are heavily screened for concerns associated with space travel, like claustrophobia, homesickness, and depression. Yet despite rigorous psychological assessment and preparation, mental health support remains just as necessary as the physical component. Dr. Marshburn explains, "An astronaut may have a payload fail, making them feel as if their life's work is all for nothing. Can you imagine the stress that would then set in? There are all sorts of other things that can go wrong, causing incredible stress and anxiety."

Dr. Marshburn has a personal story along these lines. "I was five months into my second long-duration spaceflight, with another two remaining before I returned home. While reviewing my duty assignments over my morning coffee, I got a call from CAPCOM, the NASA communication liaison between astronauts and Mission Control. 'Tom,' the message said. 'We have a private conference we need you to attend right now.' I remember looking at my two crewmates. The general consensus was, 'Well, that's not good,' so I was prepared for bad news. When I connected to the private communication channel, they had my flight surgeon on the ground and my wife on the line. They told me my mother had passed the previous night.

"Looking back on it, they used several psychological techniques to break this to me. They had already prepared a private line when the first call came up, to minimize the time between the concerning first public communication and when they were able to tell only me what had happened, instead of letting me dwell on it. We didn't have a psychologist on hand, but they knew my flight surgeon and my wife would offer the best support. They also knew what to expect from me emotionally. Mission Control relieved me from all my duties for the day, giving me free rein to contact family members. They also briefed my crewmates. All this helped my psychological response."

Dr. Marshburn has also witnessed telemedicine's power to deal with strain felt by others. "I've seen ground-based psychologists talk crewmembers through really tough moments. At times, some astronauts have run into something that really shook them. A trained psychologist or psychiatrist, on the other hand, can connect one-to-one with a person. Such communication could be possible virtually using a tablet or other device. I've even seen an expert talk down a crewmember to the point they're laughing by the end of the call. As you can imagine, this assistance will prove ever more critical as more folks go to space who aren't career astronauts, but rather, private-sector experts working off-world temporarily."

OPTIMIZING WELLNESS IN SPACE

In Chapter 11 we examine advances to optimize health. Physicians are no longer limited to treating the sick. Instead, they can help patients become healthier in every life aspect. This same work can occur in space. This is an area particularly exciting to Dr. Marshburn. "We want astronauts to be at their peak at all times. This means asking questions beyond 'are they feeling sick?' and diving into more specifics, like determining how they're sleeping, what they're eating, what their mood is, and how the events of the mission are affecting them. Such questions can be answered through a combination of telehealth and continuous monitoring. Subtle detectors, they can pick up changes before astronauts even realize something's going on."

To this point, Dr. Marshburn believes we are at the nascent stages of continuous monitoring. "I've been up in space with an accelerometer on me and a watch with EKG functionality. What we really need is to be able to monitor *many* aspects of daily life in nonintrusive ways. Naturally, we think of heart rate changes and cortisol shifts. However, current discussions also center on other factors, like urine and fecal analysis. On Earth, we sometimes do analyses of bodily waste when we think someone is sick. Now, what if we can monitor such things in real time, picking up things when they happen? This could be accomplished via a nonintrusive medical exam that automatically happens when astronauts use the bathroom. Right now, we gather data through more intrusive means, like making astronauts scan a barcode to log food and liquid intake. But we can do things better in the future."

Here's another example of nonintrusive monitoring. "What if we could use one's blinking rate as a measure of fatigue? This would lead to questions about what's making the crew tired—is it overwork, or is it something else? While this might not be the right tracking method, you do need an approach. Otherwise, you're relying on self-reporting, and astronauts typically report that they are fine even when they are completely exhausted."

DIFFERENCES BETWEEN EARTH AND SPACE TELEHEALTH

Throughout the interview, Dr. Marshburn drew close parallels between telehealth, both terrestrially and in space. Important differences exist. He explains, "On Earth, a telemedicine doctor may at some point say, 'Stop what you're doing. It's time to go to the ER.' A doctor on an airplane may need to make a similar call: 'Do we need to land to get a sick passenger help, or can we push through to our destination?' Now, in space, we typically don't have the luxury of quickly landing. Instead, telehealth doctors will be pushed to do more, to walk crews through procedures they wouldn't in traditional telehealth applications. Likewise, as humanity pushes further into space, focuses will shift. They'll be looking at radiation levels, exposure to dust on planets like Mars, and the mental health challenges of being 100 million miles from home."

HOW SPACE TELEMEDICINE WILL HELP LIFE ON EARTH

Sierra Space believes building the space economy will also enhance terrestrial life. On one hand, this will occur thanks to advances in energy and materials science. On the other, it will produce greater medical advances, such as cancer treatments developed in microgravity. Dr. Marshburn points out how telehealth systems and procedures developed for use in orbit and beyond will find earthbound applications. "Here's an illustrative example. Consider how we might handle a broken arm in space. Normally, the first thing we associate with a broken bone is performing an X-ray. But we don't have X-ray machines in space, so we'll rely on ultrasound machines. Ultrasounds perform well in detecting fractures, plus we'll have excellent handheld ultrasound units on board. Based on a telehealth doctor's review of such an ultrasound, we can immobilize the arm, treating accordingly."

Certainly, such a procedure could occur on Earth, especially for underserved populations. Dr. Marshburn continues, "Many places in the United States don't require this type of care. But think about an inner-city resident who breaks her arm. They go to the ER and check in. Then they may sit there for eight hours due to staffing problems and the hospital being overwhelmed with trauma cases. This is where telehealth breakthroughs developed for space come into play. What if that person could go to a clinic run by a nurse trained to connect to a telehealth physician? They could use an inexpensive handheld ultrasound to send the data in real time to a physician to determine their injury's extent. The nurse could then place a cast on the limb and schedule a follow-up with a doctor at a time that works for everyone."

In this scenario our patient receives treatment within perhaps 30 minutes and then follows up in a way that doesn't stress the health-care system more than necessary. That's where telehealth is headed: to the benefit of astronauts orbiting 300 miles above Earth and us who remain below.

CREATING A BETTER TOMORROW

Throughout this book you've read about telemedicine's current and future applications. From lifesaving treatment for opioid addicts seeking a fresh start to keeping astronauts fit as they develop tomorrow's technological marvels, remote care has the chance to positively affect the lives of so many.

Based on the dedication of physicians who have embraced this new way to improve their patients' health and the organizations enabling such work, people of all walks of life—but especially those who have been traditionally underserved by the legacy healthcare system—shall receive better health outcomes than they ever thought possible. All thanks to telemedicine.

QuickMD and its fast-growing team of caring doctors and tech experts have blazed a path for telehealth to make its best possible impact on the health of our nation. Now we ask a simple question to the medical establishment and to the investment community: Are you ready to join the telemedicine revolution? Your patients are waiting.

Notes

CHAPTER 1

1. Julia Shaver, "The State of Telehealth before and after the COVID-19 Pandemic," *Primary Care* 49, no. 4 (2022), https://www.ncbi.nlm.nih.gov/pmc/articles/PMC9035352/.
2. Oleg Bestsennyy, Greg Gilbert, Alex Harris, and Jennifer Rost, "Telehealth: A Quarter-Trillion-Dollar Post-COVID-19 Reality?," McKinsey and Company, July 9, 2021, https://www.mckinsey.com/industries/healthcare/our-insights/telehealth-a-quarter-trillion-dollar-post-covid-19-reality.
3. Alexis E. Carrington, "How NY Hospital Faced COVID Devastation and Came Back from the Brink," *ABC News*, March 28, 2021, https://abcnews.go.com/Health/ny-hospital-faced-covid-devastation-back-brink/story?id=76638912.
4. Vikas S. Gupta, Elizabeth C. Popp, Elisa I. Garcia, Sahar Qashqai, Christy Ankrom, Tzu-Ching Wu, and Matthew T. Harting, "Telemedicine as a Component of Forward Triage in a Pandemic," *Healthcare* 9, no. 3 (2021), https://www.sciencedirect.com/science/article/pii/S2213076421000506.
5. Owen Adams, "Never Let a Crisis Go to Waste," *Healthcare Papers* 20, no. 4 (April 2022): 4–10.
6. Yvette Brazier, "What Was Medicine Like in Prehistoric Times?," *Medical News Today*, November 2, 2018, https://www.medicalnewstoday.com/articles/323556.
7. International Hippocratic Foundation of Kos, "Hippocrates Quotes," accessed March 16, 2024, https://hippocraticfoundation.org/images/hippocrat/pdf/HIPPOCRATES_QUOTES.pdf.

8. Joshua J. Mark, "Medicine in Ancient Mesopotamia," *World History Encyclopedia*, January 25, 2023, https://www.worldhistory.org/article/687/medicine-in-ancient-mesopotamia/.

9. Evan Andrews, "7 Unusual Ancient Medical Techniques," *History*, March 27, 2023, https://www.history.com/news/7-unusual-ancient-medical-techniques.

10. Charles G. Gross, *A Hole in the Head: More Tales in the History of Neuroscience* (Cambridge, MA: MIT Press, 2009), 5.

11. "Medical Ideas in the Medieval Era," BBC, accessed March 16, 2024, https://www.bbc.co.uk/bitesize/guides/zyscng8/revision/1. See also P. N. Singer, "Galen," *Stanford Encyclopedia of Philosophy*, December 3, 2021, https://plato.stanford.edu/entries/galen/#toc.

12. Rachael Zimlich, "What Was Bloodletting All About?," *Healthline*, May 3, 2021, https://www.healthline.com/health/bloodletting#summary.

13. Ina Dixon, "Civil War Medicine: Modern Medicine's Civil War Legacy," American Battlefield Trust, October 29, 2013, https://www.battlefields.org/learn/articles/civil-war-medicine.

14. Anna Maderis Miller, "Is the House Call Doctor Coming Back?," *U.S. News and World Report*, April 14, 2015, https://health.usnews.com/health-news/patient-advice/articles/2015/04/14/is-the-house-call-doctor-coming-back.

15. Miller, "Is the House Call Doctor Coming Back?"

16. Aine Givens, "181 Rural Hospitals Have Closed since 2005—See the States That Have Been Impacted," Sidecar Health, December 1, 2021, https://sidecarhealth.com/blog/181-rural-hospitals-have-closed-since-2005-see-the-states-that-have-been-impacted.

17. Jordan Rau and Emmarie Huetteman, "Some Urban Hospitals Face Closure or Cutbacks as the Pandemic Adds to Fiscal Woes," NPR, September 15, 2020, https://www.npr.org/sections/health-shots/2020/09/15/912866179/some-urban-hospitals-face-closure-or-cutbacks-as-the-pandemic-adds-to-fiscal-woe.

18. Reid Wilson, "Americans Getting Older, New Census Figures Show," *The Hill*, June 20, 2019, https://thehill.com/homenews/state-watch/449505-americans-getting-older-new-census-figures-show/.

19. Sujata Srinivasan, "Wait Times for Primary Care Physicians Are Expected to Get Longer, but Technology May Help," Connecticut Public Radio, August 18, 2023, https://www.ctpublic.org/news/2023-08-18/wait-times-for-primary-care-physician-are-expected-to-get-worse-but-technology-might-be-able-help.

20. Oliver Kharraz, "Long Waits to See a Doctor Are a Public Health Crisis," *STAT*, May 2, 2023, https://www.statnews.com/2023/05/02/doctor-appointment-wait-times-solutions/.

21. Craig Guillot, "6 Reasons Telehealth Is Now More Important Than Ever," *HealthTech*, May 14, 2020, https://healthtechmagazine.net/article/2020/05/6-reasons-telehealth-now-more-important-ever.

22. Karolina Pogorzelska and Slawomir Chlabicz, "Patient Satisfaction with Telemedicine during the COVID-19 Pandemic—a Systematic Review," *International Journal of Environmental Research and Public Health* 19, no. 10 (May 2022), https://www.ncbi.nlm.nih.gov/pmc/articles/PMC9140408/.

23. Jessica Dudley and Iuye Sung, "What Patients Like—and Dislike—about Telemedicine," *Harvard Business Review*, December 8, 2020, https://hbr.org/2020/12/what-patients-like-and-dislike-about-telemedicine.

CHAPTER 2

1. *Seinfeld*, season 2, episode 1, "The Ex-Girlfriend," directed by Tom Cherones, aired January 23, 1991, on NBC.

2. Dan Mangan, "Most Stressful Part of Doctor's Visit: The Wait, Says Survey," CNBC, April 5, 2016, https://www.cnbc.com/2016/04/05/most-stressful-part-of-doctors-visit-the-wait-says-survey.html.

3. Brad Tuttle, "It Costs You $43 to Sit around the Doctor's Waiting Room," *Money*, October 6, 2015, https://money.com/time-money-doctor-visit-healthcare/.

4. Keith Wagstaff, "Average American Loses $43 during Each Doctor Visit," *NBC News*, October 7, 2015, https://www.nbcnews.com/business/consumer/average-american-loses-43-during-each-doctor-visit-n440136.

5. Wagstaff, "Average American Loses."

6. Susan Perry, "Should We Charge Our Doctors for Wasting Our Time in Their Office Waiting Rooms?," *MinnPost*, July 8, 2011, https://www.minnpost.com/second-opinion/2011/07/should-we-charge-our-doctors-wasting-our-time-their-office-waiting-rooms/.

7. Kelly Gooch, "ER Wait Times, by State," *Becker's Hospital Review*, February 24, 2022, https://www.beckershospitalreview.com/rankings-and-ratings/er-wait-times-by-state.html.

8. Laura Christianson, "Anatomy of a Hospital, or Why Your ER Wait Time Is So Long," *Hippo Reads*, accessed February 15, 2024, https://hipporeads.com/anatomy-of-a-hospital-or-why-your-er-wait-time-is-so-long/.

9. "As ER Wait Times Grow, More Patients Leave against Medical Advice," *KFF Health News*, accessed February 15, 2024, https://kffhealthnews.org/news/as-er-wait-times-grow-more-patients-leave-against-medical-advice/.

10. Shay Arthur, "Family Says They Spent 50 Hours Waiting for Care at Memphis Hospital; Health Officials Say Some Wait Even Longer," WREG, August 30, 2021, https://wreg.com/news/family-says-they-spent-50-hours-waiting-for-care-at-memphis-hospital-health-officials-say-some-wait-even-longer/.

11. Marisela Amador, "Quebec Health Minister Says Emergency Room Death of 86-Year-Old Woman 'Disturbing,'" CTV News Montreal, March 2, 2023, https://montreal.ctvnews.ca/quebec-health-minister-says-emergency-room-death-of-86-year-old-woman-disturbing-1.6296454.

12. Sophie Lewis, "A Woman Left the Emergency Room after Waiting for Hours: She Died That Same Day," *CBS News*, January 20, 2020, https://www.cbsnews.com/news/enlarged-heart-woman-tashonna-ward-dies-waiting-for-hours-froedtert-hospital-emergency-room/.

13. Cara Murez, "Long Emergency Room Waits May Raise Risk of Death," UPI, January 19, 2022, https://www.upi.com/Health_News/2022/01/19/emergency-room-delays-death-risk/9731642622635/.

14. Christine Sinsky, Lacey Colligan, Ling Li, Mirela Prgomet, Sam Reynolds, Lindsey Goeders, Johanna Westbrook, Michael Tutty, and George Blike, "Allocation of Physician Time in Ambulatory Practice: A Time and Motion Study in 4 Specialties," *Annals of Internal Medicine*, September 6, 2016, https://doi.org/10.7326/M16-0961.

15. Shannon Aymes, "Work-Life Balance for Physicians: The What, the Why, and the How," *Medical News Today*, September 22, 2020, https://www.medicalnewstoday.com/articles/318087.

16. U.S. Bureau of Labor Statistics, "Labor Force Statistics from the Current Population Survey: Persons at Work by Occupation, Sex, and Usual Full- or Part-Time Status," January 26, 2024, https://www.bls.gov/cps/cpsaat23.htm.

17. Indeed Editorial Team, "Guide to a Lawyer's Average Hours (with Tips for Work-Life Balance)," Indeed, January 26, 2023, https://www.indeed.com/career-advice/finding-a-job/lawyer-working-hours.

18. Duane, "Doctor Work Hours by Specialty: Which Medical Professionals Work the Most Extended Shifts?," Rockford Health System, 2022, https://www.rockfordhealthsystem.org/doctor-work-hours-by-specialty/.

19. Anupam B. Jena, "Is an 80-Hour Workweek Enough to Train a Doctor?," *Harvard Business Review*, July 12, 2019, https://hbr.org/2019/07/is-an-80-hour-workweek-enough-to-train-a-doctor.

20. Jena, "80-Hour Workweek."

21. Physician's Briefing Staff, "Almost Two-Thirds of U.S. Doctors, Nurses Feel Burnt Out at Work: Poll," *HealthDay*, March 1, 2023, https://www.healthday.com/healthpro-news/general-health/almost-two-thirds-of-u-s-doctors-nurses-feel-burnt-out-at-work-poll-2659486789.html.

22. "How Many Hours Do Nurses Work?," *Nurse Theory*, accessed March 16, 2024, https://www.nursetheory.com/how-many-hours-do-registered-nurses-work/.

23. Aurora Almendral, "The World Could Be Short of 13 Million Nurses in 2030—Here's Why," World Economic Forum, January 28, 2022, https://www.weforum.org/agenda/2022/01/health-care-nurses-attrition-mental-health-burnout/.

24. Shruthi Mahalingaiah, "POV: If You're a Doctor or Med Student Thinking about Having a Family, You May Want to Get Pregnant Sooner Rather Than Later," *Boston University Today*, January 3, 2022, https://www.bu.edu/articles/2022/doctors-may-want-to-get-pregnant-sooner/.

25. Bill Siwicki, "Report: 90% of Nurses Considering Leaving the Profession in the Next Year," *Healthcare IT News*, March 24, 2022, https://www.healthcareitnews.com/news/report-90-nurses-considering-leaving-profession-next-year.

26. Tanya Albert Henry, "Medicine's Great Resignation? 1 in 5 Doctors Plan Exit in 2 Years," American Medical Association, January 18, 2022, https://www.ama-assn.org/practice-management/physician-health/medicine-s-great-resignation-1-5-doctors-plan-exit-2-years.

CHAPTER 3

1. "Nature vs. Nurture," *Psychology Today*, accessed February 15, 2024, https://www.psychologytoday.com/us/basics/nature-vs-nurture.

2. Steven Pinker, "Why Nature and Nurture Won't Go Away," *Daedalus* 133, no. 4 (Fall 2004), https://doi.org/10.1162/0011526042365591.

3. NIH National Cancer Institute, "Genetic Testing for Inherited Cancer Susceptibility Syndromes," March 15, 2019, https://www.cancer.gov/about-cancer/causes-prevention/genetics/genetic-testing-fact-sheet.

4. Centers for Disease Control and Prevention, "Health Effects of Cigarette Smoking," October 29, 2021, https://www.cdc.gov/tobacco/data_statistics/fact_sheets/health_effects/effects_cig_smoking/index.htm.

5. Centers for Disease Control and Prevention, "Social Determinants of Health at CDC," December 8, 2022, https://www.cdc.gov/about/sdoh/index.html.

6. Johns Hopkins Medicine, "Johns Hopkins Team Outlines Ways to Integrate SDOH Data," accessed March 17, 2024, https://www.hopkinsacg.org/article/johns-hopkins-team-outlines-ways-to-integrate-sdoh-data/.
7. Amanda Nguyen, Jeroen van Meijgaard, Sara Kim, and Tori Marsh, "Mapping Healthcare Deserts: 80% of the Country Lacks Adequate Access to Healthcare," GoodRx, September 2021, https://assets.ctfassets.net/4f3rgqwzdznj/1XSl43l40KXMQiJUtl0iIq/ad0070ad4534f9b5776bc2c41091c321/GoodRx_Healthcare_Deserts_White_Paper.pdf.
8. Nguyen et al., "Mapping Healthcare Deserts."
9. Nguyen et al., "Mapping Healthcare Deserts."
10. Barnini Chakraborty, "Medical Deserts: What They Are, Where They Are, and Who They Affect," *Washington Examiner*, August 9, 2022, https://www.washingtonexaminer.com/?p=2606342.
11. Megan Leonhardt, "66% of Americans Fear They Won't Be Able to Afford Health Care This Year," CNBC, January 5, 2021, https://www.cnbc.com/2021/01/05/americans-fear-they-wont-be-able-to-pay-for-health-care-this-year.html.
12. Sarah Foster, "Survey: More Than Half of Americans Couldn't Cover Three Months of Expenses with an Emergency Fund," Bankrate, July 21, 2021, https://www.bankrate.com/banking/savings/emergency-savings-survey-july-2021/.
13. National Center for Education Statistics, "Adult Literacy in the United States," *Data Point*, July 2019, https://nces.ed.gov/pubs2019/2019179/index.asp.
14. National Center for Education Statistics, "Adult Literacy."
15. Michael T. Nietzel, "Low Literacy Levels among U.S. Adults Could Be Costing the Economy $2.2 Trillion a Year," *Forbes*, September 9, 2020, https://www.forbes.com/sites/michaeltnietzel/2020/09/09/low-literacy-levels-among-us-adults-could-be-costing-the-economy-22-trillion-a-year/?sh=5e15ca764c90.

16. Cleveland Clinic, "Here's How Fast Food Can Affect Your Body," *Health Essentials*, January 27, 2021, https://health.clevelandclinic.org/heres-how-fast-food-can-affect-your-body/.

17. Ann Wright, "Interactive Web Tool Maps Food Deserts, Provides Key Data," U.S. Department of Agriculture, May 3, 2011, https://www.usda.gov/media/blog/2011/05/03/interactive-web-tool-maps-food-deserts-provides-key-data.

18. Congressional Research Service, "Defining Low-Income, Low-Access Food Areas (Food Deserts)," *In Focus*, June 1, 2021, https://crsreports.congress.gov/product/pdf/IF/IF11841.

19. Robert C. Meisner, "Ketamine for Major Depression: New Tool, New Questions," *Harvard Health Blog*, May 22, 2019, https://www.health.harvard.edu/blog/ketamine-for-major-depression-new-tool-new-questions-2019052216673.

20. Brian D. Smedley, Adrienne Y. Stith, and Alan R. Nelson, eds., *Unequal Treatment: Confronting Racial and Ethnic Disparities in Health Care* (Washington, DC: National Academies Press, 2003), https://nap.nationalacademies.org/catalog/12875/unequal-treatment-confronting-racial-and-ethnic-disparities-in-health-care.

21. Meredith Grady and Tim Edgar, "Appendix D: Racial Disparities in Health Care: Highlights from Focus Group Findings," in Smedley, Stith, and Nelson, *Unequal Treatment*, 392–405.

22. Martha Hostetter and Sarah Klein, "Understanding and Ameliorating Medical Mistrust Among Black Americans," Commonwealth Fund, January 14, 2021, https://www.commonwealthfund.org/publications/newsletter-article/2021/jan/medical-mistrust-among-black-americans.

23. Janice Hopkins Tanne, "Patients Are More Satisfied with Care from Doctors of Same Race," *BMJ* 325, no. 7372 (2002), https://www.ncbi.nlm.nih.gov/pmc/articles/PMC1124573/.

24. Lindsay Carlton, "Patients Prefer Doctors of Same Race and Ethnicity, Study Finds," *Verywell Health*, November 19, 2020, https://www.verywellhealth.com/patient-provider-preference-race-ethnicity-5088173.

25. *Freakonomics*, episode 6, "Are Barbershops the Cutting Edge of Healthcare Delivery?," hosted by Bapu Jena, produced by Jessica Wapner, aired September 9, 2021, https://freakonomics.com/podcast/are-barbershops-the-cutting-edge-of-healthcare-delivery/.
26. Tara Parker-Pope, "Should You See a Female Doctor?," *New York Times*, August 14, 2018, https://www.nytimes.com/2018/08/14/well/doctors-male-female-women-men-heart.html.
27. Kyle J. Tobler, John Wu, Ayatallah M. Khafagy, Bruce D. Pier, Saioa Torrealday, Laura Londra, "Gender Preference of the Obstetrician Gynecologist Provider," *Obstetrics and Gynecology* 127 (May 2016): 43S.
28. Ryan Boetel, "Doctors Flee New Mexico—and More Are Expected to Follow," *Albuquerque Journal*, February 4, 2023, https://www.abqjournal.com/news/local/doctors-flee-new-mexico-and-more-are-expected-to-follow/article_8ed1d0f3-a009-5de2-820c-d2f0637c60b6.html.
29. Boetel, "Doctors Flee New Mexico."
30. American Public Transportation Association, "Public Transportation Facts," accessed February 16, 2024, https://www.apta.com/news-publications/public-transportation-facts/.
31. American Hospital Association, "Social Determinants of Health Series: Transportation and the Role of Hospitals," November 15, 2017, https://www.aha.org/ahahret-guides/2017-11-15-social-determinants-health-series-transportation-and-role-hospitals.

CHAPTER 4

1. Computer History Museum, "Timeline of Computer History," accessed February 16, 2024, https://www.computerhistory.org/timeline/computers/.
2. Larry Abramson, "Classroom Computers, Another Legacy of Steve Jobs," NPR, October 8, 2011, https://www.npr.org/2011/10/09/141186979/computers-in-class-another-legacy-of-steve-jobs.

3. Phil Edwards, "In Memoriam: AOL CDs, History's Greatest Junk Mail," *Vox*, May 12, 2015, https://www.vox.com/2015/5/12/8594049/aol-free-trial-cds.

4. Caitlin Dewey, "A Complete History of the Rise and Fall—and Reincarnation!—of the Beloved '90s Chatroom," *Washington Post*, October 30, 2014, https://www.washingtonpost.com/news/the-intersect/wp/2014/10/30/a-complete-history-of-the-rise-and-fall-and-reincarnation-of-the-beloved-90s-chatroom/.

5. Hayley Matthews, "The History of Online Dating: A Timeline from Paper Ads to Websites," DatingAdvice.com, January 24, 2024, https://www.datingadvice.com/online-dating/history-of-online-dating.

6. Hayley Matthews, "The History of Match.com (from 1993 to Today)," *DatingAdvice.com*, December 15, 2022, https://www.datingnews.com/apps-and-sites/history-of-match/.

7. Harley Hahn and Rick Stout, *The Internet Yellow Pages* (New York: McGraw-Hill, 1996).

8. Jeremy Salvucci, "What Was the Dot-Com Bubble and Why Did It Burst?," *TheStreet*, January 12, 2023, https://www.thestreet.com/dictionary/dot-com-bubble-and-burst.

9. Ken Yeung, "LinkedIn Is 10 Years Old Today: Here's the Story of How It Changed the Way We Work," *TNW*, May 5, 2013, https://thenextweb.com/news/linkedin-10-years-social-network.

10. Konstantin Guericke, "How LinkedIn Broke Through," *Bloomberg*, April 9, 2006, https://www.bloomberg.com/news/articles/2006-04-09/how-linkedin-broke-through.

11. Niraj Chokshi, "Myspace, Once the King of Social Networks, Lost Years of Data from Its Heyday," *New York Times*, March 19, 2019, https://www.nytimes.com/2019/03/19/business/myspace-user-data.html.

12. Pew Research Center, "Internet, Broadband Fact Sheet," January 31, 2024, https://www.pewresearch.org/internet/fact-sheet/internet-broadband/.

13. Jon Cowling, "A Brief History of Skype—the Peer to Peer Messaging Service," DSP, February 8, 2016, https://content.dsp.co.uk/history-of-skype.

14. Ben Gilbert and Sarah Jackson, "Steve Jobs Unveiled the First iPhone 16 Years Ago—Look How Primitive It Seems Today," *Business Insider*, January 9, 2023, https://www.businessinsider.com/first-phone-anniversary-2016-12?op=1.

15. IEEE Technology Navigator, "Mediated Reality," accessed February 17, 2024, https://technav.ieee.org/topic/mediated-reality.

16. Cale Guthrie Weissman, "A Brief Timeline of How Slack Took Over the Modern Workplace in 8 Years," *Fast Company*, June 20, 2019, https://www.fastcompany.com/90366968/slack-timeline-how-it-went-from-glitch-to-nyse-in-8-years.

17. Georgia Wells, Jeff Horwitz, and Deepa Seetharaman, "Facebook Knows Instagram Is Toxic for Teen Girls, Company Documents Show," *Wall Street Journal*, September 14, 2021, https://www.wsj.com/articles/facebook-knows-instagram-is-toxic-for-teen-girls-company-documents-show-11631620739.

18. Jim Merithew, "Mark Zuckerberg's Letter to Investors: 'The Hacker Way,'" *Wired*, February 1, 2012, https://www.wired.com/2012/02/zuck-letter/.

19. Jennifer Rankin and Angelique Chrisafis, "'A State Scandal': Calls for Inquiry into Macron's Links to Uber Lobbying," *The Guardian*, July 11, 2022, https://www.theguardian.com/news/2022/jul/11/uber-files-france-calls-for-inquiry-into-emmanuel-macron-links-to-lobbying.

20. Madeline Farber, "Uber Reportedly Had a Secret 'Hell' Program to Track Lyft Drivers," *Fortune*, April 13, 2017, https://fortune.com/2017/04/13/uber-lyft-hell/.

21. Matt McFarland, "Uber Self-Driving Car Operator Charged in Pedestrian Death," *CNN Business*, September 18, 2020, https://www.cnn.com/2020/09/18/cars/uber-vasquez-charged/index.html.

22. Merithew, "Mark Zuckerberg's Letter."

23. Steve Banker, "Tesla Has the Highest Accident Rate of Any Auto Brand," *Forbes*, December 18, 2023, https://www.forbes.com/sites/stevebanker/2023/12/18/tesla-has-the-highest-accident-rate-of-any-auto-brand/?sh=4c5369ea2894.

24. Andrei Nedelea, "NHTSA Probing Tesla for Two More Driver Assistance System-Related Crashes," *Inside EVs*, December 29, 2022, https://insideevs.com/news/628720/nhtsa-probes-tesla-fsd-new-crashes/.

25. Shoshana Zuboff, *The Age of Surveillance Capitalism: The Fight for a Human Future at the New Frontier* of *Power* (New York: PublicAffairs, 2019).

26. Joanna Kavenna, "Shoshana Zuboff: 'Surveillance Capitalism Is an Assault on Human Autonomy,'" *The Guardian*, October 4, 2019, https://www.theguardian.com/books/2019/oct/04/shoshana-zuboff-surveillance-capitalism-assault-human-automomy-digital-privacy.

27. Naomi Diaz, "18 Hospitals, Health Systems Facing Lawsuits for Healthcare Data-Sharing," *Becker's Hospital Review*, April 26, 2023, https://www.beckershospitalreview.com/healthcare-information-technology/9-hospitals-health-systems-facing-lawsuits-for-healthcare-data-sharing.html.

28. Art Van Zee, "The Promotion and Marketing of OxyContin: Commercial Triumph, Public Health Tragedy," *American Journal of Public Health* 99, no. 2 (February 2009), https://ajph.aphapublications.org/doi/pdf/10.2105/AJPH.2007.131714.

29. Julian Borger, "Hillbilly Heroin: The Painkiller Abuse Wrecking Lives in West Virginia," *The Guardian*, June 25, 2001, https://www.theguardian.com/world/2001/jun/25/usa.julianborger.

30. Mary Pat Flaherty and Gilbert M. Gaul, "Experimentation Turns Deadly for One Teenager," *Washington Post*, October 21, 2003, https://www.washingtonpost.com/archive/politics/2003/10/21/experimentation-turns-deadly-for-one-teenager/c4061cf7-52fd-4731-b82d-ca95f3bd260f/.

31. "Pharmacist Nailed for Online Drug Sales," *ABC News*, June 17, 2024, https://abcnews.go.com/GMA/story?id=127762&page=1.

32. Jan Philipp Wilhelm, "The Unbelievable Story of Paul le Roux," *DW*, July 6, 2020, https://www.dw.com/en/from-programmer-to-gangster-boss-the-unbelievable-story-of-paul-le-roux/a-54047877.

33. Federal Emergency Management Agency, "COVID-19 Emergency Declaration," March 14, 2020, https://www.fema.gov/press-release/20210318/covid-19-emergency-declaration.

34. Christi A. Grimm, "Geographic Disparities Affect Access to Buprenorphine Services for Opioid Use Disorder," U.S. Department of Health and Human Services Office of Inspector General, January 2020, https://oig.hhs.gov/oei/reports/oei-12-17-00240.pdf.

35. American Medical Association, "Medications to Treat Opioid Use Disorder (MOUD)," accessed February 17, 2024, https://www.ama-assn.org/topics/medications-treat-opioid-use-disorder-moud. See also Tanya Albert Henry, "New Rules Enable Telemedicine Treatment for Opioid-Use Disorder," American Medical Association, March 12, 2024, https://www.ama-assn.org/delivering-care/overdose-epidemic/new-rules-enable-telemedicine-treatment-opioid-use-disorder.

36. William C. Goedel, Aaron Shapiro, Magdalena Cerdá, Jennifer W. Tsai, Scott E. Hadland, and Brandon D. L. Marshall, "Association of Racial/Ethnic Segregation with Treatment Capacity for Opioid Use Disorder in Counties in the United States," *JAMA Network Open* 3, no. 4 (2020), https://jamanetwork.com/journals/jamanetworkopen/fullarticle/2764663.

37. Utsha Khatri, Corey S. Davis, Noa Crawczyk, Michael Lynch, Justin Berk, and Elizabeth A. Samuels, "These Key Telehealth Policy Changes Would Improve Buprenorphine Access While Advancing Health Equity," *Health Affairs*, September 11, 2020, https://www.healthaffairs.org/content/forefront/these-key-telehealth-policy-changes-would-improve-buprenorphine-access-while-advancing.

38. Meaghan McCabe, "Whitehouse, Portman Laud Proposed Rule to Continue Telehealth Treatment for Opioid Use Disorder," Sheldon Whitehouse, December 16, 2022, https://www.whitehouse.senate.gov/news/release/whitehouse-portman-laud-proposed-rule-to-continue-telehealth-treatment-for-opioid-use-disorder.

39. Jason Langendorf, "What Can We Expect from the CARA 3.0 Bill?," *Treatment Magazine*, April 12, 2021, https://treatmentmagazine.com/what-can-we-expect-from-the-cara-3-0-bill/.

CHAPTER 5

1. American Hospital Association, "Fast Facts on US Hospitals, 2021," January 2021, https://www.aha.org/system/files/media/file/2021/01/Fast-Facts-2021-table-FY19-data-14jan21.pdf.
2. Randall Hallett and Michael Ashley, *Vibrant Vulnerability: Mastering Philanthropy for Today and Tomorrow's Healthcare CEOs* (Independently published, 2023).
3. Randall Hallett, Zoom interview by the authors, 2023. All other quotations from Hallett in this chapter come from this interview.
4. Tim van Beisen and Todd Johnson, "Ambulatory Surgery Center Growth Accelerates: Is Medtech Ready?," Bain and Company, September 23, 2019, https://www.bain.com/insights/ambulatory-surgery-center-growth-accelerates-is-medtech-ready/.
5. American Hospital Association, "Massive Growth in Expenses and Rising Inflation Fuel Financial Challenges for America's Hospitals and Health Systems," April 22, 2022, https://www.aha.org/guidesreports/2022-04-22-massive-growth-expenses-and-rising-inflation-fuel-continued-financial.
6. Milken Institute School of Public Health, "The Growing Cost of Aging in America, Part 1: An Aging Population and Rising Health Care Costs," April 6, 2018, https://onlinepublichealth.gwu.edu/resources/cost-of-aging-healthcare/.
7. Sonny B. Bal, "An Introduction to Medical Malpractice in the United States," *Clinical Orthopaedics and Related Research* 467, no. 2 (February 2009), https://journals.lww.com/clinorthop/fulltext/2009/02000/an_introduction_to_medical_malpractice_in_the.4.aspx.

8. Hoag Levins, "Hospital Consolidation Continues to Boost Costs, Narrow Access, and Impact Care Quality," Penn LDI, January 19, 2023, https://ldi.upenn.edu/our-work/research-updates/hospital-consolidation-continues-to-boost-costs-narrow-access-and-impact-care-quality/.
9. Thomas Waldrop and Emily Gee, "How States Can Expand Health Care Access in Rural Communities," Center for American Progress, February 9, 2022, https://www.americanprogress.org/article/how-states-can-expand-health-care-access-in-rural-communities/.
10. Stephanie Hughes, "While Undergraduate Enrollment Stabilizes, Fewer Students Are Studying Health Care," *Marketplace*, February 2, 2023, https://www.marketplace.org/2023/02/02/while-undergraduate-enrollment-stabilizes-fewer-students-are-studying-health-care/.
11. Tait D. Shanafelt, Colin P. West, Lotte N. Dyrbye, Mickey Trockel, Michael Tutty, Hanhan Wang, Lindsey E. Carlasare, and Christine Sinsky, "Changes in Burnout and Satisfaction with Work-Life Integration in Physicians During the First 2 Years of the COVID-19 Pandemic," *Mayo Clinic Proceedings* 97, no. 12 (December 2022): 2248–2258.
12. Rashid L. Bashshur, Gary W. Shannon, Brian R. Smith, Dale C. Alverson, Nina Antoniotti, William G. Barsan, Noura Bashshur, et al., "The Empirical Foundations of Telemedicine Interventions for Chronic Disease Management," *Telemedicine and e-Health* 20, no. 9 (September 3, 2014): 769–800; Edwin A. Takahashi, Lee H. Schwamm, Opeolu M. Adeoye, Olamide Alabi, Eiman Jahangir, Sanjay Misra, and Carolyn H. Still, "An Overview of Telehealth in the Management of Cardiovascular Disease: A Scientific Statement from the American Heart Association," *Circulation* 146, no. 25 (December 2022), https://doi.org/10.1161/CIR.0000000000001107.
13. Hossein Hatami, Niloofar Deravi, Bardia Danaei, Moein Zangiabadian, Amir Hashem Shahidi Bonjar, Ali Kheradmand, and Mohammad Javad Nasiri, "Tele-medicine and Improvement of Mental Health Problems in COVID-19 Pandemic: A Systematic Review," *International Journal of Methods in Psychiatric Research* 31, no. 3 (September 2022), https://doi.org/10.1002/mpr.1924.

14. Zara Greenbaum, "The Stigma That Undermines Care," American Psychological Association, June 2019, https://www.apa.org/monitor/2019/06/cover-opioids-stigma.

15. Julia Adler-Milstein, Joseph Kvedar, and David W. Bates, "Telehealth among US Hospitals: Several Factors, Including State Reimbursement and Licensure Policies, Influence Adoption," *Health Affairs* 33, no. 2 (February 2014), https://doi.org/10.1377/hlthaff.2013.1054.

16. David Marcozzi, Brendan Carr, Aisha Liferidge, Nicole Baehr, and Brian Browne, "Trends in the Contribution of Emergency Departments to the Provision of Hospital-Associated Health Care in the USA," *International Journal of Social Determinants of Health and Health Services* 48, no. 2 (2018): 267–288.

17. David Kohn, "University of Maryland School of Medicine Study Finds That Nearly Half of U.S. Hospital-Associated Medical Care Comes from Emergency Rooms," University of Maryland School of Medicine, October 20, 2017, https://www.medschool.umaryland.edu/news/2017/university-of-maryland-school-of-medicine-study-finds-that-nearly-half-of-us-hospital-associated-medical-care-comes-from-emergency-rooms.html.

18. Lisa Jo Rudy and Pilar Trelles, "Why Autism Diagnoses Have Soared," *Verywell Health*, October 24, 2023, https://www.verywellhealth.com/when-did-autism-start-to-rise-260133.

19. Autism Research Institute, "Autism Prevalence Rises to 1 in 54," March 27, 2020, https://autism.org/autism-prevalence-1-in-54.

20. Natalie A. Caine, Jon O. Ebbert, Laura E. Raffals, Lindsey M. Philpot, Karna K. Sundsted, Amanda E. Mikhail, Meltiady Issa, Anne A. Schletty, and Vijay H. Shah, "A 2030 Vision for the Mayo Clinic Department of Medicine," *Mayo Clinic Proceedings* 97, no. 7 (July 2022), https://doi.org/10.1016/j.mayocp.2022.02.010; "How the Mayo Clinic Built Its Reputation as a Top Hospital," *Knowledge at Wharton*, August 28, 2018, https://knowledge.wharton.upenn.edu/article/mayo-clinics-secret-success/.

CHAPTER 6

1. Tiffany Casper, "5 Tips to Keep Burnout at Bay," Mayo Clinic Health System, October 8, 2021, https://www.mayoclinichealthsystem.org/hometown-health/speaking-of-health/5-tips-to-keep-burnout-at-bay.
2. American Medical Association, "Measuring and Addressing Physician Burnout," May 3, 2023, https://www.ama-assn.org/practice-management/physician-health/measuring-and-addressing-physician-burnout.
3. Tait D. Shanafelt, Colin P. West, Lotte N. Dyrbye, Mickey Trockel, Michael Tutty, Hanhan Wang, Lindsey E. Carlasare, and Christine Sinsky, "Changes in Burnout and Satisfaction with Work-Life Integration in Physicians During the First 2 Years of the COVID-19 Pandemic," *Mayo Clinic Proceedings* 97, no. 12 (December 2022): 2248–2258.
4. Oliver Whang, "Physician Burnout Has Reached Distressing Levels, New Research Finds," *New York Times*, September 29, 2022, https://www.nytimes.com/2022/09/29/health/doctor-burnout-pandemic.html.
5. Whang, "Physician Burnout."
6. National Academy of Medicine, *Taking Action against Clinician Burnout: A Systems Approach to Professional Well-Being* (Washington, DC: National Academies Press, 2019).
7. Danielle Fallon-O'Leary, "Work-Life Integration Is the New Work-Life Balance: Is Your Team Ready?," U.S. Chamber of Commerce, accessed February 17, 2024, https://www.uschamber.com/co/grow/thrive/work-life-integration-vs-work-life-balance.
8. Shanafelt et al., "Changes in Burnout."
9. Shanafelt et al., "Changes in Burnout."
10. Shanafelt et al., "Changes in Burnout."
11. Shanafelt et al., "Changes in Burnout."
12. Liselotte N. Dyrbye, Wayne Sotile, Sonja Boone, Colin P. West, Litjen Tan, Daniel Satele, Jeff Sloan, Mick Oreskovich, and Tait Shanafelt, "A Survey of U.S. Physicians and Their Partners Regarding the Impact of Work-Home

Conflict," *Journal of General Internal Medicine* 29, no. 1 (January 2014): 155–161; Ariela L. Marshall, Liselotte N. Dyrbye, Tait D. Shanafelt, Christine A. Sinsky, Daniel Satele, Mickey Trockel, Michael Tutty, and Colin P. West, "Disparities in Burnout and Satisfaction with Work-Life Integration in U.S. Physicians by Gender and Practice Setting," *Academic Medicine* 95, no. 9 (September 2020): 1435–1443; Daniel S. Tawfik, Tait D. Shanafelt, Liselotte N. Dyrbye, Christine A. Sinsky, Colin P. West, Alexis S. Davis, Felice Su, et al., "Personal and Professional Factors Associated with Work-Life Integration among US Physicians," *JAMA Network Open* 4, no. 5 (2021), https://jamanetwork.com/journals/jamanetworkopen/fullarticle/2780406.

13. Shanafelt et al., "Changes in Burnout."

14. Sara Berg, "Pandemic Pushes U.S. Doctor Burnout to All-Time High of 63%," American Medical Association, September 15, 2022, https://www.ama-assn.org/practice-management/physician-health/pandemic-pushes-us-doctor-burnout-all-time-high-63.

15. Keith Ferrazzi and Mike Clementi, "The Great Resignation Stems from a Great Exploration," *Harvard Business Review*, June 22, 2022, https://hbr.org/2022/06/the-great-resignation-stems-from-a-great-exploration.

16. Arianne Cohen, "How to Quit Your Job in the Great Post-pandemic Resignation Boom," *Bloomberg*, May 10, 2021, https://www.bloomberg.com/news/articles/2021-05-10/quit-your-job-how-to-resign-after-covid-pandemic.

17. Christina Pazzanese, "'I Quit' Is All the Rage: Blip or Sea Change?," *Harvard Gazette*, October 20, 2021, https://news.harvard.edu/gazette/story/2021/10/harvard-economist-sheds-light-on-great-resignation/.

18. Juliana Kaplan, "The Psychologist Who Coined the Phrase 'Great Resignation' Reveals How He Saw It Coming and Where He Sees It Going," *Business Insider*, October 2, 2021, https://www.businessinsider.com/why-everyone-is-quitting-great-resignation-psychologist-pandemic-rethink-life-2021-10?op=1.

19. Kaplan, "Psychologist Who Coined."

20. Kaplan, "Psychologist Who Coined."
21. "Ayurvedic Medicine," *Weil*, accessed February 18, 2024, https://www.drweil.com/health-wellness/balanced-living/wellness-therapies/ayurvedic-medicine/.
22. Robert C. Meisner, "Ketamine for Major Depression: New Tool, New Questions," *Harvard Health Blog*, May 22, 2019, https://www.health.harvard.edu/blog/ketamine-for-major-depression-new-tool-new-questions-2019052216673.

CHAPTER 7

1. Danielle Campagne, "Fracture-Dislocation of the Midfoot (Lisfranc Injury)," *Merck Manual*, December 2022, https://www.merckmanuals.com/professional/injuries-poisoning/fractures/fracture-dislocation-of-the-midfoot-lisfranc-injury.
2. National Institute on Drug Abuse, "Heroin Research Report," June 2018, https://nida.nih.gov/publications/research-reports/heroin/overview.
3. National Institute on Drug Abuse, "Naloxone Drug Facts," January 2022, https://nida.nih.gov/publications/drugfacts/naloxone.
4. U.S. Food and Drug Administration, "Information about Medication-Assisted Treatment (MAT)," May 23, 2023, https://www.fda.gov/drugs/information-drug-class/information-about-medication-assisted-treatment-mat.
5. Adam Viera, Daniel J. Bromberg, Shannon Whittaker, Bryan M. Refsland, Milena Stanojlović, Kate Nyhan, and Frederick L. Altice, "Adherence to and Retention in Medications for Opioid Use Disorder among Adolescents and Young Adults," *Epidemiologic Reviews* 42, no. 1 (2020): 41–56.
6. See the PwrdBy website, at https://pwrdby.com.
7. See the Brave website, at https://www.brave.coop.

CHAPTER 8

1. "A Quarter-Century of Changes: Ads We Can't Get out of Our Heads," *USA Today*, accessed February 18, 2024, https://usatoday30.usatoday.com/money/top25-ads.htm.

2. "Woman Who Fell, Then Starred in 'I Can't Get Up' TV Ads Dies," *Deseret News*, August 2, 1997, https://www.deseret.com/1997/8/2/19326983/woman-who-fell-then-starred-in-i-can-t-get-up-tv-ads-dies.

3. Dewey Webb, "Catch a 'Fallen' Star," *Phoenix New Times News*, December 19, 1990, http://web.archive.org/web/20140219150201/https:/www.phoenixnewtimes.com/1990-12-19/news/catch-a-fallen-star/.

4. Webb, "Catch a 'Fallen' Star."

5. Webb, "Catch a 'Fallen' Star."

6. Noelle Greenway, "A Brief History behind the Phrase: 'I've Fallen and I Can't Get Up!,'" *Medical Alert Advice*, March 1, 2024, https://www.medicalalertadvice.com/articles/a-brief-history-behind-the-phrase-ive-fallen-and-i-cant-get-up/.

7. Webb, "Catch a 'Fallen' Star."

8. "I've Fallen and I Can't Get Up," *Know Your Meme*, accessed February 18, 2024, https://knowyourmeme.com/memes/ive-fallen-and-i-cant-get-up--3.

9. Association of Schools Advancing Health Professions, "Emerging Clinical Role of Wearables," March 22, 2021, https://www.asahp.org/trends-test-1/2021/03/22/american-rescue-plan-becomes-law-dmxak-rex7j-58bst-ybcsr-jm8jz-2yym2.

10. Jamie Ballard, "Many Americans Can't Go More Than a Few Hours without Their Smartphones," YouGov, June 25, 2018, https://today.yougov.com/technology/articles/21053-smartphone-habits-millennials-boomers-gen-x.

11. Samsung, "View Your Step Count in Samsung Health," accessed February 19, 2024, https://www.samsung.com/us/support/answer/ANS00080925/.

12. Tim Hardwick, "iPhone 14: How Crash Detection Works and How to Turn It Off," *MacRumors*, September 16, 2022, https://www.macrumors.com/how-to/iphone-14-disable-car-crash-detection/.
13. Cristina Alexander, "The Apple Watch Series 8's Crash Detection Already Saved Someone's Life," *Digital Trends*, October 28, 2022, https://www.digitaltrends.com/mobile/apple-watch-series-8-crash-detection-already-saved-someones-life/.
14. Joanna Stern, "'The Owner of This iPhone Was in a Severe Car Crash'—or Just on a Roller Coaster," *Wall Street Journal*, October 9, 2022, https://www.wsj.com/articles/the-owner-of-this-iphone-was-in-a-severe-car-crashor-just-on-a-roller-coaster-11665314944.
15. Georgia Worrell, "Apple's Faulty 'Crash Detection' Feature Dials 911 When Skiers Take a Tumble," *New York Post*, January 14, 2023, https://nypost.com/2023/01/14/apples-crash-detection-dials-911-when-skiers-take-a-tumble/.
16. Andrew Liszewski, "False 911 Calls Skyrocket during Bonnaroo as the iPhone Mistakes Dancing for Car Crashes," *Gizmodo*, June 26, 2023, https://gizmodo.com/iphones-false-911-calls-bonnaroo-android-uk-999-1850576151.
17. Jon Porter and Nick Statt, "Google Completes Purchase of Fitbit," *The Verge*, January 14, 2021, https://www.theverge.com/2021/1/14/22188428/google-fitbit-acquisition-completed-approved.
18. Meghan Holohan, "This Woman's Fitbit Didn't Simply Encourage Her to Walk—It Saved Her Life," *Today*, April 6, 2017, https://www.today.com/health/how-fitbit-device-could-actually-save-your-life-t110058.
19. Holohan, "This Woman's Fitbit."
20. James Stables, "In-Depth: Fitbit's Continuous Afib Tracking Feature Explained," *Wareable*, June 2, 2022, https://www.wareable.com/fitbit/fitbits-continuous-afib-tracking-explained-8817.

21. Carlos A. Morillo, Amitava Banerjee, Pablo Perel, David Wood, and Xavier Jouven, "Atrial Fibrillation: The Current Epidemic," *Journal of Geriatric Cardiology* 14, no. 3 (March 2017), https://www.ncbi.nlm.nih.gov/pmc/articles/PMC5460066/.

22. Shay O'Connor, "New Orleans Man Says a Fitbit Device Saved His Life; Now He's Alerting Others to Mind Their Health," *WDSU News*, May 4, 2023, https://www.wdsu.com/article/new-orleans-man-says-a-fitbit-device-saved-his-life-now-hes-alerting-others-to-mind-their-health/43785965.

23. For more information, see the Oura Ring website at https://ouraring.com.

24. Harvard Medical School Division of Sleep Medicine, "Why Sleep Matters: Benefits of Sleep," accessed February 19, 2024, https://sleep.hms.harvard.edu/education-training/public-education/sleep-and-health-education-program/sleep-health-education-41.

25. Renee Cherry, "I Tried the Oura Ring for 2 Months—Here's What to Expect from the Tracker," *Shape*, January 13, 2021, https://www.shape.com/fitness/gear/tech/oura-ring-review.

26. Cherry, "I Tried the Oura Ring."

27. Mark Gurman, "Apple Makes Major Progress on No-Prick Blood Glucose Tracking for Its Watch," *Bloomberg*, February 22, 2023, https://www.bloomberg.com/news/articles/2023-02-22/apple-watch-blood-glucose-monitor-could-revolutionize-diabetes-care-aapl.

28. Mayo Clinic Diseases and Conditions, "Diabetes," accessed February 19, 2024, https://www.mayoclinic.org/diseases-conditions/diabetes/symptoms-causes/syc-20371444.

29. Steven D. Bagley and Michael Ashley, *Never Alone: A Man's Companion Guide to Grief* (Independently published, 2021).

30. Helen Ouyang, "Your Next Hospital Bed Might Be at Home," *New York Times Magazine*, January 26, 2023, https://archive.is/p3mKl#selection-403.0-403.39.

31. Ouyang, "Your Next Hospital Bed."

32. Ouyang, "Your Next Hospital Bed."

33. Ouyang, "Your Next Hospital Bed."

CHAPTER 9

1. Rainforest Trust, "The Peruvian Amazon," accessed February 19, 2024, https://www.rainforesttrust.org/our-impact/success-stories/the-peruvian-amazon/.

2. Jillian Kubala, "What Is Ayahuasca? Experience, Benefits, and Side Effects," *Healthline*, December 16, 2022, https://www.healthline.com/nutrition/ayahuasca.

3. Ira Israel, "What to Expect During an Ayahuasca Ceremony," *mindbodygreen*, February 20, 2020, https://www.mindbodygreen.com/articles/what-to-expect-during-an-Ayahuasca-ceremony.

4. National Center for Complementary and Integrative Health, "Traditional Chinese Medicine: What You Need to Know," accessed February 19, 2024, https://www.nccih.nih.gov/health/traditional-chinese-medicine-what-you-need-to-know.

5. Emily A. Vogels, Risa Gelles-Watnick, and Navid Massarat, "Teens, Social Media and Technology, 2022," Pew Research Center, August 10, 2022, https://www.pewresearch.org/internet/2022/08/10/teens-social-media-and-technology-2022/.

6. Katie Steinmetz, "Teens Are Over Face-to-Face Communication, Study Says," *Time*, September 10, 2018, https://time.com/5390435/teen-social-media-usage/.

7. Centers for Disease Control, "New CDC Data Illuminate Youth Mental Health Threats during the COVID-19 Pandemic," March 31, 2022, https://www.cdc.gov/media/releases/2022/p0331-youth-mental-health-covid-19.html.

8. Brightline, "FAQ," accessed March 26, 2024, https://www.hellobrightline.com/faq/.

9. Sam Hubley, Sarah B. Lynch, Christopher Schneck, Marshall Thomas, and Jay Shore, "Review of Key Telepsychiatry Outcomes," *World Journal of Psychiatry* 6, no. 2 (2016): 269–282.

10. Mayo Clinic "Cognitive Behavioral Therapy," March 16, 2019, https://www.mayoclinic.org/tests-procedures/cognitive-behavioral-therapy/about/pac-20384610.

11. David Grodberg, "Children's Disruptive Behavior Can Sap Work Productivity: We Have a Solution," Brightline, July 27, 2021, https://www.hellobrightline.com/blog/disruptive-behavior-disorder-solution/.

12. Grodberg, "Children's Disruptive Behavior"; John M. Salsman, Zeeshan Butt, Paul A. Pilkonis, Jill M. Cyranowski, Nicholas Zill, Hugh C. Hendrie, Mary Jo Kupst, et al., "Emotion Assessment Using the NIH Toolbox," *Neurology* 80, no. 11, suppl. 3 (March 12, 2013): S76–S86.

13. Naomi Allen, "It's Time for Corporate America to Address the Youth Mental Health Crisis," *Fast Company*, July 19, 2022, https://www.fastcompany.com/90770039/its-time-for-corporate-america-to-address-the-youth-mental-health-crisis.

14. Kenneth C. Nash, Zoom interview by the authors, 2023. All other quotations from Nash in this chapter come from this interview.

15. World Justice Project, "rAInbow: Chatbot to Support Victims of Domestic Abuse," accessed February 19, 2024, https://worldjusticeproject.org/world-justice-challenge-2021/rainbow-chatbot-support-victims-domestic-abuse.

CHAPTER 10

1. Foley & Lardner, "Telemedicine and Digital Health," accessed March 17, 2024, https://www.foley.com/sectors/health-care-life-sciences/telemedicine-digital-health/.

2. Kyle Y. Faget, Zoom interview by the authors, 2023. All other quotations from Faget in this chapter come from this interview.
3. Emily Olsen, "Report: COVID-19 Accelerates Health Tech Investment in 2021," *MobiHealthNews*, December 8, 2021, https://www.mobihealthnews.com/news/report-covid-19-accelerates-health-tech-investment-2021.
4. Heather Landi, "SoftBank Leads Mental Health Startup Cerebral's $300M Round, Propelling Valuation to $4.8B," *Fierce Healthcare*, December 8, 2021, https://www.fiercehealthcare.com/tech/softbank-leads-mental-health-startup-cerebral-s-300m-round-propelling-valuation-to-4-8b.
5. Nathaniel M. Lacktman, "2023 Forecast for Digital Health Startups and Telemedicine Law," *Foley Blogs*, January 10, 2023, https://www.foley.com/insights/publications/2023/01/2023-forecast-digital-health-startups-telemedicine/.
6. Chris Larson, "Troubled Digital Mental Health Startup Cerebral Lays Off More Than 1,000 Employees," *Behavioral Health Business*, October 24, 2022, https://bhbusiness.com/2022/10/24/troubled-digital-mental-health-startup-cerebral-lays-off-more-than-1000-employees/.
7. American Hospital Association, "New Report Highlights Financial Challenges Facing Hospitals That Are Jeopardizing Access to Care," September 15, 2022, https://www.aha.org/special-bulletin/2022-09-15-new-report-highlights-financial-challenges-facing-hospitals-are.

CHAPTER 11

1. Institute for Functional Medicine, "The Functional Medicine Approach," accessed February 19, 2024, https://www.ifm.org/functional-medicine/what-is-functional-medicine/.
2. For more information, see the Cleveland Clinic Center for Functional Medicine website at https://my.clevelandclinic.org/departments/functional-medicine.

3. Sam Lavis, Zoom interview by the authors, 2023. All other quotations from Lavis in this chapter come from this interview.

4. Mercey Livingston and Kim Wong-Shing, "Best Continuous Glucose Monitors of 2024," *CNET*, January 26, 2024, https://www.cnet.com/health/medical/best-continuous-glucose-monitors/.

5. Ayanna Redwood-Crawford, "The Oura Ring Is a $300 Sleep Tracker That Provides Tons of Data: But Is It Worth It?," *New York Times*, September 14, 2023, https://www.nytimes.com/wirecutter/reviews/oura-ring-sleep-tracker/.

6. Cara Murez, "Telemedicine's Popularity Has Risen during Pandemic," *U.S. News and World Report*, November 8, 2022, https://www.usnews.com/news/health-news/articles/2022-11-08/telemedicines-popularity-has-risen-during-pandemic.

7. Shira H. Fischer, Zachary Predmore, Elizabeth Roth, Lori Uscher-Pines, Matthew Baird, and Joshua Breslau, "Use of and Willingness to Use Video Telehealth through the COVID-19 Pandemic," *Health Affairs* 41, no. 11 (November 2022), https://doi.org/10.1377/hlthaff.2022.00118. See also the RAND American Life Panel website, at https://alpdata.rand.org/.

8. Fischer et al., "Use of and Willingness."

9. Roni Caryn Rabin, "Racial Inequities Persist in Health Care Despite Expanded Insurance," *New York Times*, August 29, 2021, https://www.nytimes.com/2021/08/17/health/racial-disparities-health-care.html.

10. Medtronic, "The Rise of—and Demand for—Telehealth Equity," June 29, 2022, https://news.medtronic.com/The-rise-and-demand-of-telehealth-equity.

11. Medtronic, "Rise of."

12. Shira H. Fischer, "Americans' Willingness to Use Video Telehealth Has Risen during COVID-19 Pandemic," RAND, November 7, 2022, https://www.rand.org/news/press/2022/11/07/index1.html.

13. A. M. Totten, M. S. McDonagh, and J. H. Wagner, "The Evidence Base for Telehealth: Reassurance in the Face of Rapid Expansion

during the COVID-19 Pandemic," AHRQ white paper, May 14, 2020, https://effectivehealthcare.ahrq.gov/products/telehealth-expansion/white-paper.

14. Totten, McDonagh, and Wagner, "Evidence Base for Telehealth."

CHAPTER 12

1. Sierra Space, "The Future of Commercial Space Stations: LIFE Habitat," accessed February 20, 2024, https://www.sierraspace.com/space-destinations/life-inflatable-space-habitat/.
2. Jeff Foust, "Sierra Space Describes Long-Term Plans for Dream Chaser and Inflatable Modules," *Space News*, June 28, 2023, https://spacenews.com/sierra-space-describes-long-term-plans-for-dream-chaser-and-inflatable-modules/.
3. National Aeronautics and Space Administration, "Astronaut Biography: Thomas H. Marshburn," May 2022, https://www.nasa.gov/wp-content/uploads/2023/07/marshburn-thomas.pdf.
4. "US Astronauts Complete Spacewalk to Replace Antenna after Debris Scare," *ABC News*, December 2, 2021, https://www.abc.net.au/news/2021-12-03/us-astronauts-complete-spacewalk-antenna-debris-scare/100671552.
5. Sierra Space, "Sierra Space Bolsters Human Spaceflight Center and Astronaut Training Academy Team," December 1, 2022, https://www.sierraspace.com/newsroom/press-releases/sierra-space-bolsters-human-space-flight-center-and-astronaut-training-academy-team/.
6. Thomas H. Marshburn, Zoom interview by the authors, 2023. All other quotations from Marshburn in this chapter come from this interview.

Index

B

C

D

E

F

G

J

K

L

M

N

O

P

Q

R

S

T

U

V

W

Y

Z

About the Authors

CHRIS ROVIN serves as the vice president of operations and physician management for QuickMD. Since 2021, Chris has been directly responsible for scaling up the number of telemedicine doctors working for the company by more than 10 times in just two years.

Following his education at the University of Michigan, he entered a career in brain tumor research. Chris then felt the pull to focus on opportunities to unite tech and medicine, creating WeSearch, the first charity crowdfunding platform to combine donors and vital innovative research struggling to find funding.

Chris earned his MBA degree at Pepperdine and then entered the medical device industry as head of product at PwrdBy. His interest in medical devices led to his next major product, which would bring together the future QuickMD team.

Chris has contributed to multiple books and articles on nonprofit management and health technology, including *Likeable Business: Why Today's Consumers Demand More and How Leaders Can Deliver.*

JARED SHEEHAN serves as the chief innovation officer at QuickMD.

After graduating from Miami University with a BS degree in accounting and environmental science, Jared worked for Deloitte Consulting. He then found a way to combine his passions for technology and improving medical care as president of Neeka Health.

Jared received an MS degree in environmental science and policy from Johns Hopkins University and subsequently served as chief executive officer of PwrdBy, a social impact incubator that created next-generation technologies for nonprofits, hospitals, and mission-driven organizations.

For over a decade, Jared has cofounded technology-driven companies supporting various social impact industries and has advised corporations on corporate social responsibility and sustainable practices.

Jared has been featured in *Forbes*, is a TEDx speaker, and writes for numerous publications, including *Becker's Hospital Review*, *Modern Healthcare*, *NonProfit PRO*, and those of the Colorado Institute for Social Impact and LA Tech4Good. Jared also serves as the treasurer of the Youth Business Alliance and is an advisor with LA Tech4Good, the Big Wild, and the AI for Good Foundation.

TALIB OMER, MD, founded QuickMD and serves as one of its medical directors and a board member. Dr. Omer's vision with QuickMD is to ensure that quality healthcare is accessible, affordable, and convenient for all Americans, regardless of where they live and their socioeconomic circumstances.

Dr. Omer was inspired to become a doctor by his father, a primary care doctor in Germany, and his older brother, who is an associate professor of pediatrics at Baylor. After receiving his MD and PhD degrees from the Albert-Ludwigs University in Freiburg, Germany, he ultimately completed his residency training in emergency medicine at Yale University.

Dr. Omer remains an active and board-certified ER physician in a level 1 trauma center, where he has an academic appointment as associate professor of clinical emergency medicine from the University of Southern California (USC). There, Dr. Omer is also advancing state-of-the-art care for conditions such as traumatic injuries, acute strokes, and heart attacks.

Dr. Omer has also published and presented extensive research, with keynotes and lectures at USC's Keck School of Medicine, UCLA, Kern Medical Center, American College of Emergency Physicians, Council of Residency Directors in Emergency Medicine, AHIP's Consumer Experience and Digital Health Forum, and more.

MICHAEL ASHLEY began his writing career as a newspaper reporter and playwright before transitioning to Hollywood to work for the head of the literary department at Creative Artists Agency. He also served as a screenwriter for Disney, where he sold the treatment for the hit Halloween movie *Girl vs. Monster*. A former screenwriting professor, Michael has written more than 50 books on many subjects, especially cutting-edge technology.

An in-demand professional speaker, Michael is a columnist for *Forbes*, *Entrepreneur*, and *Becker's Hospital Review*. His prolific work has been featured in *Fox Sports*, *Entertainment Weekly*, the *National Examiner*, the United Nations' *ITU News*, the *Orange County Business Journal*, the *Austin Daily Herald*, *Yahoo! Finance*, *HuffPost*, and the *Boston Herald*.